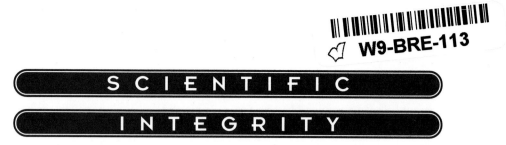

SCIENTIFIC
INTEGRITY

An Introductory Text with Cases

Francis L. Macrina

Professor and Chair
Department of Microbiology and Immunology
Medical College of Virginia
Virginia Commonwealth University
Richmond, Virginia

ASM Press • Washington, D.C.

Publisher's Note:

Scientific Integrity: an Introductory Text with Cases is intended to serve as a text for courses and seminars on scientific research and integrity. The text is not meant in any way to serve as a set of guidelines, rules, or statements officially endorsed by the American Society for Microbiology.

The case studies used throughout this text are hypothetical and are not intended to describe any actual organization or real person, living or dead. The opinions in the text, expressed or implied, are those of the authors and do not represent official policies of the American Society for Microbiology.

Copyright © 1995   American Society for Microbiology
1325 Massachusetts Avenue, N.W.
Washington, DC 20005

Library of Congress Cataloging-in-Publication Data

Macrina, Francis L.
  Scientific integrity: an introductory text with cases / Francis
L. Macrina.
      p.   cm.
  Includes bibliographical references and index.
  ISBN 1-55581-069-1
  1. Research—Moral and ethical aspects.   2. Medical sciences—
Research—Moral and ethical aspects.   3. Integrity.   I. Title.
  Q180.55.M67M33   1995
  174'.95072—dc20   94-46226
                                                                      CIP

To Mary

Contents

Preface

This textbook grew from a course in Scientific Integrity which I began developing at Virginia Commonwealth University in the mid-1980s. The course was originally offered on a noncredit basis and encompassed scientific skills such as verbal and written communication, as well as topics related to conduct in science. Then, in 1989, the National Institutes of Health mandated that trainees with certain types of federal support receive formal instruction in the responsible conduct of science. This marked a period of rapid evolution in the course content in order to thoroughly cover topics relevant to scientific integrity. I asked other experts to join me in this teaching endeavor, and our Scientific Integrity course (formalized in 1991) has been offered as a one-credit-hour course ever since.

My teaching colleagues joined me in writing this book because we discovered that there was no suitable teaching text. There were a number of essay collections and monographs about scientific integrity, but none covered the full range of topics we felt essential to teaching graduate students in the biomedical, life sciences and chemistry. Another problem with available readings was the lack of a valuable teaching tool: the case study that linked basic information to specific examples, thereby illustrating important points. Coupling background knowledge with practical applications makes teaching the principles of scientific integrity more challenging and interesting for both students and instructors. We have included case studies that draw from the material presented in each chapter to illustrate the diversity of issues that have been identified as scientific integrity and to give students the opportunity to develop the concepts presented by reasoned practice.

We have relied heavily on the case study approach in this book and in our teaching. Students discuss model cases in our course. They apply their knowledge along with their personal and professional values to solve problems. We have found this method of teaching the principles of scientific integrity to be effective. The students enjoy discussing cases and it's clear they learn from them. It's fun for the teachers as well, and we often find ourselves learning new things right along with our students.

Our text is aimed at pre- and postdoctoral trainees in the biomedical and natural sciences. It also will be useful to individuals who train or practice in related scientific fields. Although the precepts of scientific integrity can be taught at different academic levels, our text is geared for graduate biomedical trainees, preferably those who have some exposure to the research laboratory. Usually, this means students who are at least beginning the second year of graduate study. There is a culture, language, and mind set that accompanies life in the research laboratory which is not revealed in the classroom setting. We believe that prior laboratory exposure greatly facilitates teaching the principles of scientific integrity. Most importantly it gives the students a basis for identifying with the cases and provides them with a preview of the range of the issues they are likely to encounter in practicing scientific research.

In short, this is a book that covers a variety of topics related to the conduct of scientific investigation, but it is *not* a rulebook for the scientist. We discuss guidelines and policies, standards, and codes because we want our readers to be aware that the ultimate resolution of many of these issues is influenced by both written policies and normative standards. We also offer guidelines concerning some of the acceptable ways to approach these challenges. Yet, the values of the individual scientist take on major importance in conducting scientific research. Scientists continually make judgments and decisions about their research. Whether the issue is the timely release of experimental materials to a colleague or decisions about authorship on a manuscript, personal and professional standards and values certainly come into play. Thus, definitive, unambiguous advice on dealing with these complex issues cannot be taught in textbooks. There are many acceptable possibilities.

We refer throughout the text to guidelines and policy documents that are germane to the conduct of scientific research. This illuminates and emphasizes important aspects of research activities that fall under written mandate of one sort or another. We did not attempt to assemble a compendium of all such relevant material. This would be impractical on several grounds, not the least of which is the rapid state of change of many such documents. However, we have provided in the appendices guidance on where various relevant documents have been compiled or can be located.

Our goal is to plant the seed of inquiry in our readers' minds so that they will continually seek out current guideline and policy documents. Lifelong learning is as much a part of scientific integrity as it is of any rigorous scientific discipline.

Francis L. Macrina
Richmond, Virginia

Acknowledgments

I would like to thank all of the reviewers of the earlier drafts of the manuscript. Their comments and criticisms helped us improve the book significantly. These reviewers include:

Kenneth De Ville, Ph.D., J.D., East Carolina University; Susan Gottesman, Ph.D., National Institutes of Health; James R. Broach, Ph.D., Princeton University; Kenneth I. Berns, M.D., Cornell University Medical College; Vincent A. Fischetti, Ph.D., Rockefeller University; Christine McHenry, M.D., University of Cincinnati; Alan N. Schechter, M.D., National Institutes of Health; Stanley G. Korenman, M.D., University of California, Los Angeles; J. W. Bennett, Ph.D., Tulane University: Thomas J. Lindell, Ph.D., The University of Arizona; David L. Goodstein, Ph.D., California Institute of Technology; and Kathryn V. Holmes, Ph.D., Uniformed Services University of the Health Sciences.

Any shortcomings in the book are, of course, the responsibility of the authors.

Special thanks are extended to those who helped us with ideas for writing some of the cases, for information on the federal regulations and other issues related to scientific integrity, and for general inspiration and help in ways too numerous to mention: Claudia Blair, Robert Buery, Hank Burke, Herbert Chermside, Jan Chlebowski, Scott Diehl, Paul Ferrara, Cindy Fuchs, Michael Kalichman, Norma Kenyon, Frank Leftwich, Robert Martin, Lawrence Rhoades, Andrew Rowan, Howard Schachman, Peter Vallentyne, Glenn Van Tuyle, Alison Weiss, Lynn Willis, Rodney Welch, and James Zwolenik.

The author thanks Patrick Fitzgerald, Director of ASM Press, for his advice, patience, and encouragement. He was a vital part of this project.

Thanks to Mary, Laurel, and Frank Macrina for their understanding, and for love and support. And thanks to my parents and mentors.

Note to Students and Instructors

Many of the topics covered in teaching scientific integrity lend themselves to the case study approach and we have found its use in our course to be instructive and enjoyable. Our suggestions for making the case study approach work well are presented here and are intended to aid both students and instructors. Additional examples of case studies in responsible scientific conduct may be found in the books by Korneman and Shipp (1994), Bailar *et al.* (1990), and Penslar (1994).

How To Use End-of-Chapter Case Studies

Short case studies are found at the conclusion of all but the introductory chapter and are designed for classroom discussion. Most of these depict a "real life" scenario and contain a narrative script with fictitious characters. Others cover issues for thought and discussion. The typical case study is 200 to 400 words in length and can be read aloud in a few minutes. Most have been tested in our course.

A few that are only modestly challenging have been placed at the beginning of each set of chapter cases. Using these cases to get started is recommended. These are designed to acquaint the student and instructor with the process of case discussion and resolution using examples which lack the complexity of later cases in the set.

On the first day of class, we distribute a printed copy of all the cases, and groups of cases are assigned to students for each of the subsequent class sessions. These students will be called on to discuss the case on an assigned date. The students select cases they are interested in from their assigned set of cases (relevant to each day's topic). Small groups of two to three seem to work best in implementing this strategy. Students can decide among themselves on a few cases and prepare for their presentation. By assigning a case set in advance of the class, students have a chance to think about their arguments, and also have time to do research or consultation on the topic if needed. They may, for example, want to consult relevant guidelines or policy documents. Although most cases don't require research, they may not work as well when students have not been exposed to a graduate research environment.

Sets of cases should be assigned to small student groups ahead of the class in which the corresponding chapter material will be covered. The students should select cases they wish to discuss and then individually lead the discussion in the class period. Guidelines for leading discussion are given below. Our class periods are either 1 or 1½ hours, and we allow for a minimum of 20 minutes to discuss two to four cases.

A student leading the discussion begins by reading the case aloud in class. He or she then acts as the moderator for the rest of the discussion of that particular case. Discussion is aided by a seating arrangement that allows everyone in the classroom to see one another (e.g., seating around a conference table, or arranging chairs into a circle or semicircle). Typical classroom seating arrangements with students facing the front of the room make it difficult for everyone to see who's talking during open discussions and this inconvenience can dampen group participation. Case discussions work well in small classrooms, optimally with fewer than 20 but not more than 25 students.

Effective student participation is central to the process. The instructor should only serve as a facilitator, contributing when clarification is needed, when discussion bogs down, or when closure on a case is appropriate. The student reads the case and presents his or her impressions, identifying the issues and suggesting a possible solution. The classroom is then open to discussion where students air their views on the topic (without having more than one person talking at once). The instructor or student moderator may have to act as a peacekeeper. Sometimes disputes arise; discussions can become animated and even intense. If the dialogue becomes emotional, insulting or inappropriate comments should not be allowed. Ad hominem comments are totally unacceptable and discussants should be cautioned against their use.

Short cases are designed to encourage the discussants to think critically as they analyze and solve the problem at hand. For many cases, this will mean dissecting the facts of the case and separating the relevant issues from those that are irrelevant. Cases will evoke uncertainties and ambiguities, and the discussion can begin by having students ask questions about the case. If something needs clarification or explanation, it should be provided by the student leading the discussion where possible or by the instructor when help is needed.

The cases are specifically designed to allow discussants to apply their knowledge and personal standards to problems encountered in doing scientific research. Discussion should often lead to one or more acceptable solutions to the same problem. This is important to remember in bringing cases to closure. Much of the time a consensus answer will not emerge. There may be several "right answers," all of which are acceptable. In proposing solutions, discussants should always be able to arrive at a position that can be defended. Answers may be ranked by merit as part of the case discussion, but usually this is not necessary. A solution is valid as long as it is legal and doesn't violate what the discussants view as acceptable norms and standards, written or otherwise.

Acceptable solutions to the problem posed by the case always must be in compliance with standards related to global considerations (e.g., issues related to plagiarism or human rights). Solutions to cases always need to be examined to be sure they cannot be misinterpreted. In other words, they should not contain any "loopholes." Although there may be several acceptable solutions or answers to the problem, there always are clear "wrong answers." Such things as violations of specific standards, guidelines, or rules and regulations fall into this category as well as solutions that are inconsistent with the written or unwritten ethical standards for scientific conduct generally accepted by the profession.

The case reader should evaluate the quality and quantity of the class discussion and bring the case to closure at the appropriate time. Summarizing the discussion helps to do this. Any opposing points of view should be adequately represented in the summary. Occasionally, there may be students who are uncomfortable with the outcomes reached. If this happens, the instructor should urge continued discussion outside of the classroom with him or her or with the student's mentor.

In summary, case discussion should foster critical thinking as the discussants examine and apply their personal and professional values. The process is one of self-discovery as students formulate answers based on their values and knowledge of professional standards. The application of relevant guidelines, codes, and policies should be brought into play whenever possible. One final note on case resolution. We have deliberately omitted discussing the possible "answers" to the cases. Cases often have multiple acceptable solutions. Hashing over multiple acceptable answers runs the risk of assigning specific values to the various possibilities, which we feel is not desirable. Further, conflict resolution has too many subtleties to presuppose that simplistic answers can be applied universally to behaviors that have elements in common with a case study. The process of solving the case studies is key to learning from them. Finally, each case will have readily apparent "wrong answers," and we anticipate that these will be obvious.

Extended Case Studies and Surveys

Appendix II contains a different style of case study. It is longer and usually describes a more complex scenario. The required response is usually guided by specific questions or by a request to complete a written exercise. We call this format the extended case. A number of these appear in Appendix II and explore in depth specific chapter topics. We have successfully used these extended cases to form the basis of a writing assignment for our course. Students have been required to select four cases and write a response of one to two typewritten single-spaced pages per case. In effect this becomes a "term paper" upon which part of the course grade can be based.

Appendix I contains some surveys which we have found to be useful teaching tools. As with the short cases, we assign these surveys to small groups of students on the first day of class. They collect the completed response sheets from their classmates on an assigned date, collate the data, and present an analysis of the results. Printed response sheets corresponding to each survey are provided by the instructor. Anonymity is a requisite in these surveys and this is stressed in the instructions printed on the response sheet. The assignment includes the date by which the rest of the class must turn in their responses to the students conducting the survey. A date on which the results of the survey will be discussed in class is also set. Class time is reserved during a relevant session for discussion of the survey results. The student survey-takers then collate the data and prepare a handout or overhead transparency for class presentation of the results. Discussion is led by the student survey-takers and class participation is encouraged. For example, responses to questions that displayed considerable disparity can be explored. Invariably, there will be questions where a significant number of students strongly agree with a point of view, while a similar number strongly disagree with it. Discussion of such differing points of view can be valuable. In that sense, we have found that these exercises have provided some of the same benefits as the short case discussions. Class debate is lively and students come to recognize and appreciate differing points of view on issues related to scientific conduct and training.

REFERENCES

Bailar, J., M. Angell, S. Boots, E. Myers, N. Palmer, M. Shipley, and P. Woolf. 1990. *Ethics and Policy in Scientific Publication.* Editorial Policy Committee, Council of Biology Editors, Bethesda, MD.

Korneman, S. G., and A. C. Shipp. 1994. *Teaching Responsible Conduct of Research Through a Case Study Approach.* Association of American Medical Colleges, Washington, D.C.

Penslar, R. L. (ed.) 1994. *Research Ethics: Cases and Materials.* Indiana University Press, Bloomington.

1 | Scientific Integrity

Francis L. Macrina

Integrity in Science

What do we mean by "integrity in science"? Science is knowledge that comes from the collection, organization, and interpretation of facts. It is the search for truth. Integrity paints an image of solid moral principles. People of integrity are morally upright, honest, fair, and sincere. When applied to concepts or information, integrity conjures images of wholeness, totality, and completeness. The practice of science is thus limited to people of integrity.

That assertion in today's world sparks heated debate: science and scientists are under intense public scrutiny. Headlines, news shows, books, and magazine articles speak of "stolen viruses," "science under siege," "falsified results," "scapegoats," "whistleblowers," and "scientific hoaxes." Do scientists really lie, cheat, and steal? The public wants to know and the media has responded with zealous and aggressive investigations of alleged scientific misconduct.

Most scientists argue that the incidence of misconduct in science is very low, but a frank assessment of the problem is warranted. Federal agencies and panels of experts who have studied the issue have called for further research and reliable data. Indeed, investigations of alleged incidents along with cases of proven misconduct have led some scientists to admit that the image of science has been justifiably tarnished. Scientific and lay communities alike have recognized that science includes some practitioners who are capable of reprehensible behavior.

Clearly, scientists make honest mistakes and these must not be confused with, or interpreted as, misconduct. As with any professionals, scientists are fallible, impressionable, impulsive, and subjective. They sometimes fall prey to self-deception and may rationalize in ways that mislead themselves and others. Terms like "sloppy science" are frequently used to describe such behavior, but the distinctions between "sloppy science" and "scientific misconduct" are nebulous. Identifying and dealing with behavior that falls between these two distinct forms of conduct has indeed been difficult. However, deliberate deception in scientific research is different and constitutes scientific fraud. Governmental organizations have tended to avoid this term in favor of "scientific misconduct." The word "fraud" has specific legal meaning which has complicated prosecution of alleged incidents.

The formal education of a scientist stretches over a period of years punctuated by academic degrees, but informal learning is ongoing. When scientists assume their professional roles, this creates a framework for practicing science. The knowledge that guides scientists' decisionmaking processes is obviously interwoven with their moral principles, yet they learn about standards of conduct for scientific research in varying ways. Some take formal courses in the subject. Others study the written standards of conduct of agencies and scientific societies, or follow institutional documents that codify certain aspects of responsible conduct. Still others learn by observing their mentors or other respected scientists.

Scientists continuously apply standards to the conduct of their research. Sometimes the process is second nature and the issues being handled are taken for granted. Unacceptable behavior is readily apparent and can have significant negative effects on scientists' abilities to function professionally. Some simple questions can illuminate this perspective. Have accepted practices for record keeping and data storage been followed? Under what circumstances is it appropriate to use humans or animals in research? What regulations and policies apply to such experimentation? What are the rules that govern conflict of interest in scientific research? How do matters of intellectual property affect scientists? What are the considerations of process, courtesy, and confidentiality that guide scientific peer review? What guidelines or policies exist for assigning authorship on scientific papers?

Awareness of and adherence to accepted standards of conduct is the basis of scientific integrity. The relative merits of some standards (e.g., authorship criteria) have been the subject of much debate. Distinguishing acceptable from unacceptable practices is not always easy. Norms in some areas are not well established or are evolving.

Whether written or unwritten, standards for doing research provide the foundation for training scientists to properly conduct science. Betrand Russell's argument makes a cogent point. He believes that we trace "the evils of the world" to moral defects and lack of intelligence. We know little about eliminating moral defects and unethical behavior. On the other hand, we can improve intelligence by teaching relevant material. So, we seek to improve intelligence rather than improving morals. Russell's argument is relevant to the teaching of scientific integrity. Both practicing scientists and scientists-in-training must continuously examine the subject, play a role in the refinement of existing standards, and contribute to the development of needed standards. This is a starting point for pursuing those activities.

Scientific Misconduct

During the past three decades, the existence of misconduct in science has been recognized by the scientific community, investigated by governmental agencies, and publicized to society. The biomedical sciences have suffered the brunt of the negative publicity. The scientific community, however, has not been particularly organized in its analysis of or response to scientific misconduct. In the United States, the two principal funding agencies of the biomedical and natural sciences, the National Institutes of Health (NIH) and the National Science Foundation (NSF), began responding with new or extended initiatives in the 1980s. The NIH, an agency of the U.S. Public Health Service (USPHS), expanded its Office of Scientific Integrity, which eventually was renamed the Office of Research Integrity. The NSF reaffirmed the role of its Office of Inspector General in matters of scientific misconduct. Both of these agencies undertook the refinement of their definitions of scientific misconduct. Since the mid-1980s there have been numerous versions presented, discussed, and revised. At this writing, both the USPHS and the NSF have definitions in force.

The USPHS holds that:

> "Misconduct" or "Misconduct in Science" means fabrication, falsification, plagiarism, or other practices that seriously deviate from those that are commonly accepted

within the scientific community for proposing, conducting, or reporting research. It does not include honest error or honest differences in interpretations or judgments of data. (*Federal Register* **54**:32446–32451, August 8, 1989)

This particular definition evolved from one immediate predecessor, published in 1986. Three modified versions were proposed in the early 1990s, but were not implemented. A revised definition is expected to replace the current one.

The NFS definition states that:

Misconduct means fabrication, falsification, plagiarism or other serious deviation from accepted practices in preparing, carrying out, or reporting results from activities funded by NSF, or retaliation of any kind against a person who reported or provided information about suspected or alleged misconduct and who has not acted in bad faith. (*Federal Register* **56**:22286–22290, May 14, 1991)

This definition was revised from one originally published in 1987.

Some scholarly societies, universities, and research institutes have prepared their own definitions of scientific misconduct. Often, the USPHS or NSF definition has been directly adopted or modified for such purposes.

These two definitions provide content for a general discussion of the various definitions, and revisions of definitions, that have been published from different agencies and institutions in the past decade. First, there is a consensus that includes the terms "falsification, fabrication, and plagiarism." Falsification means tampering with results, fabrication means making up results, and plagiarism means stealing someone else's ideas. Reduction to these seemingly common denominators makes things pretty simple. Honestly searching for and telling the truth is the essence of scientific integrity. But, the language beyond the consensus core often differs. Both USPHS and NSF definitions talk about accepted research practices and warn against seriously deviating from them; such serious deviations constitute scientific misconduct. However, guidance on "accepted practices" and "serious deviations" is not readily available. Sometimes practices are written down and deviation from them is implied. There is arguably an unwritten but widely practiced code of conduct of scientific investigation and scientists know serious deviations when they see them. Scientific misconduct definitions have thus created controversy and caused arguments and confusion in the scientific and legal communities. Some of the confusion has been damaging, because one person's accepted practice may be unacceptable to another. And, even when difference of opinion is legitimate, the specter of scientific misconduct may turn such a disagreement into a high-stakes game.

The controversy associated with the publication of definitions of scientific misconduct does offer promise as scientists, their institutions, and their funding agencies begin to think more concretely about "accepted practices" and "serious deviations" in research. Long overdue general relevant concepts are being identified and clarified in the process. The NIH example conveys that scientists may disagree about the interpretation of results. It even says that scientists may make errors in their work. However, it goes on to clarify that neither of these things is scientific misconduct. The NSF definition considers the "whistleblower": the person who reports an alleged incident of misconduct. It makes retaliation against that person ("who has not acted in bad faith") an act of scientific misconduct.

Other discussion about the definitions of scientific misconduct has involved using the word "misconduct" instead of "fraud." David Goodstein has compared research fraud to civil fraud (4). In pursuing civil fraud there must be a plaintiff to file charges against the defendant. The plaintiff brings the case to court and must prove five points: (1) false representation has occurred; (2) the defendant knew the representation was false; (3) belief in the misrepresentation was promoted; (4) the plaintiff believed the misrepresentation within reason; and (5) damage resulted from the misrepresentation. Goodstein points out that in science there is little preoccupation with the fourth and fifth points (5). Thus far, these issues have been of minor consequence in proving scientific fraud. Does this justify abandoning the term "fraud" and using only "misconduct" when talking about science? As mentioned earlier, government agencies have done exactly this, but their decision has not been universally supported. For example, Howard Schachman recounts that the legalistic preference to use the word "misconduct" instead of "fraud" in science had its basis in the burden of having to prove intent and injury as is the case with civil fraud (10). He contends that the word "misconduct" engenders vagueness and that it "invites over-expansive interpretation."

Nevertheless, governmental agencies have avoided use of the word "fraud" in order to preclude getting bogged down in proving "intent to deceive" as well as in demonstrating evidence of injury in prosecution of various investigations. Goodstein (4) considers use of the word "fraud" in the regulations at his university. He argues that "the Caltech rules assume that in such offenses as faking data, plagiarism, and misappropriation of ideas, intent to deceive is manifest." Because scientific misconduct proceedings are not usually held in a court of law, that assumption may be appropriate, at least for the time being.

Another contentious issue concerns the phrase "other serious deviation," which is present in both the NIH and NSF definitions, although proposals to eliminate it have been made. A National Academy of Sciences (NAS) panel report proposed a definition in 1992 which did not include this phrase (9). The panel's report argued that such phraseology was vague and created confusion about classifying misconduct in the context of scientific research. Specifically, the panel expressed concern about an interpretation of this clause that might result in someone being accused of scientific misconduct based on "their use of novel or unorthodox research methods." Others have strongly argued for the retention of the "other serious deviation" phrase (3). The NAS panel report invoked a category of "other misconduct" beyond that of scientific misconduct involving incidents that "1) do not require expert knowledge to resolve these complaints and, 2) should be governed by mechanisms that apply to all institutional members, not just those who receive government research awards." In general, the NAS report holds that not all types of unacceptable behavior are unique to the scientific arena. Arguments which run counter to this position have been offered (3). For example, plagiarism is not unique to science and transgressions involving the theft of intellectual property are covered by civil law, yet plagiarism is a specific component of the definition of scientific misconduct. Donald Buzzelli argues that in such cases federal funding agencies have an enforcement role that protects the integrity of the research process and its funding mission (3). This leads to his central argument that some actions must be classified as scientific misconduct irrespective of whether they are covered by general laws or regulations or whether they are unique to science and scientific research. Examples of misconduct which Buzzelli places into the "other serious deviation" category include tampering and vandalism. In contrast, the NAS panel report contends that such transgressions are "subject to generally applicable legal and social penalties" and that "recognized legal and institutional procedures should be in place to address complaints and to discourage behavior involving forms of misconduct that are not unique to the research process" (9). The report specifically mentions personal and sexual harassment, misuse of funds, gross negligence, violations of governmental research regulations, and misuse of humans and animals in research. Some, if not all, of these categories may or may not be unique to the laboratory or research setting and only time and experience will help resolve these issues. Buzzelli (3) proposes that the principal criterion for resolution of such issues is whether or not the actions "do serious harm to science." He points out that the NAS panel report actually takes a similar position by invoking scientific misconduct where such actions "directly damage the integrity of the research process."

Definitions of misconduct have become part of scientific culture. Any institution receiving research support from NIH is required to have a policy in place for dealing with scientific misconduct, which must obviously be defined in the process. Nonetheless, misconduct definitions have been controversial and vigorously debated. This debate is likely to continue for some time and the revision and replacement of definitions at the federal level is anticipated. Current definitions need to be part of the working vocabulary of the scientist, and scientists need to be part of debate that will establish a background of knowledge that will ultimately allow definitions to work. Specifically, the methods of science and the styles and behavior of scientists create a confusing mix that makes the conceptualization of "accepted practices" impracticable. That difficulty, however, should not stifle dialogue, search for knowledge, and, most importantly, education in the principles of scientific integrity.

Perceptions of Science and Scientists

Scientists use the scientific method when they do research. Consideration of the scientific method in relation to the concept of scientific integrity is illuminating. How do scientists perceive their practice of science and how is it perceived by those outside of the scientific community? Nobel laureate J. Michael Bishop described his ideas on the problems facing science in recent times (12). He claims that science is underfunded, underappreciated, and under the scrutiny of a public that is unschooled in its fundamentals. This has generated an atmosphere of "fear, bewilderment, disdain...and...mistrust." Scientists facing the difficult possibility of winning grant funds, justifying their use of animals in biomedical research, and explaining to the lay public why the "war on cancer" still hasn't been won have a challenging task defending the cause of science and their expenditure of public funds. Further, the public perceives science as the definitive vehicle for uncovering truth and becomes confused when scientists disagree or argue with one another. It is difficult for the lay person to understand how scientific facts can be disputed. Yet, one federal agency definition of scientific misconduct expects that scientists will have "honest differences in interpretations of judgments of data" and that "honest error" in science does occur. The public has difficulty with the possibility that the scientific method may give erroneous results. In advertising, for example, there seems to be no greater virtue than the claim that some product was "scientifically tested" or, better yet, "scientifically proven to achieve results." The public likes to believe that the "scientific truth" is the last word. But when new facts cause scientists to change their previous interpretations and conclusions, the effect on the public is disquieting. By way of example, consider the reporting of toxicologic and safety aspects of drugs and foods. People react with sarcasm and disbelief as they read that what was good for them last year is now being reported as a potential carcinogen. The very nature of scientific investigation makes the accumulation of new information and the interpretation of existing data subject to periodic, if not regular, change.

Scientists recognize that science normally works in these ways. In general, people outside of science do not have this same appreciation of the process. Disagreements, errors, and new interpretations of results are often reported by the media, and it is easy for such reports to be misinterpreted. The discussion and debate of emerging or evolving scientific knowledge can be seen as confusion and even accusation. Thus, the integrity of science may be called into question by the people who observe it. Compounding this problem is a publicly held stereotype described by Goodstein, which he calls the "Myth of the Noble Scientist."

> The Noble Scientist is supposed to be more virtuous and
> upright than ordinary mortals, impervious to the baser hu-

man drives, such as personal ambition, and, of course, incapable of misbehaving in even the smallest way.... Because science is a very human activity, hypocrisies and misrepresentations are built into the way we do it. For example, every scientific paper is written as if that particular investigation were a triumphant procession from one truth to another. All scientists who perform research, however, know that every scientific experiment is chaotic—like war. You never know what is going on; you cannot usually understand what the data mean. But in the end, you figure out what it was all about and then, with hindsight, you write it up describing it as one clear and certain step after the other. This is a kind of hypocrisy, but it is deeply embedded in the way we do science. We are so accustomed to it that we don't even regard it as a misrepresentation anymore.... The Myth of the Noble Scientist serves us poorly precisely because it obscures the distinction between harmless minor hypocrisies and real fraud.

When the scientific method is applied, it will inherently reflect the individuality of the people doing the work. The questions asked, the tools used to get the answers, and, most importantly, the interpretation of results will be unique to the researchers. Creativity and intellect play an important role in these activities, as do work ethic and dedication, personal bias, and honesty. There is also peer pressure in science. Sometimes scientists follow trends: they use in vogue methods and make interpretations based on widely accepted beliefs.

In summary, the human behavior that is part of scientific research may influence how that research is done. The effects of behavior patterns may vary, as may the degree to which their perception by scientists or the public is gauged as "good" or "bad." Sorting out these effects is likely to be a challenge for scientists and a source of confusion for nonscientists. Failure to appreciate the element of human behavior in the performance of scientific research can lead to misunderstandings that may erroneously confuse actions of individuals as inappropriate behavior.

Scientific Method

It is commonly accepted that scientific research proceeds according to "the" scientific method which begins with the identification of a problem. In such an organized and systematically applied scientific method, some gap in knowledge is first identified and relevant questions are posed. Existing information is studied and a hypothesis—a prediction or an "educated guess"—is designed to explain perceived facts. The creation of a hypothesis is often reliant upon the scientist's use of inductive reasoning in forming a belief after considering many facts or observations. This individual approach underscores the process as a human activity. It will be affected by the knowledge, opinions, foibles, and biases of the investigator. Sir Peter Medawar holds that a hypothesis should proceed with some notion of expected results of the experiment (7). Hypotheses are subjective and those which are restrictive are generally considered to serve the investigator better than those which are permissive. Broad "guesses" are not likely to provide much insight when they are tested.

Hypotheses are subject to experimental testing using technologies and observational methods selected by the scientist. Historically, this has usually meant the decision of an individual, but the complexity and collaborative nature of current scientific research, especially biomedical research, has frequently resulted in these decisions being made collectively. In either event, again the process is profoundly human in nature—a blending of "gut feeling" and intellect is used to make decisions. Information is gathered, analyzed, and interpreted in the process of testing a hypothesis. Results may support or refute a hypothesis; a hypothesis cannot be proven. Indeed, hypotheses can only be falsified or disproven. Further testing of specific hypotheses (or their derivatives) which strengthens their support leads to the genesis of a theory. Theories take into account a strongly supported hypothesis or set of hypotheses and, in doing so, represent a broadly accepted understanding of some natural concept. Since they are based on supported hypotheses, it follows that theories can also eventually be disproven; the ultimate proof of a theory cannot be achieved. When hypotheses are not supported, the results that contribute to such a conclusion are often used to refine or to construct other hypotheses, and the process begins anew. A hypothesis which has been unequivocally rejected based on the interpretation of experimental evidence can provide the inspiration for a new hypothesis which will survive the test of repeated attempts to reject it. The value of a hypothesis resides in its ability to stimulate additional thinking and further research, much more so than whether or not it was initially correct.

In practice, the scientific method does not often progress in such a well-defined manner. Scientific papers may read like paragons of logic. They may describe cleverly crafted experimental approaches applied in the most timely and compelling ways. But, in keeping with Goodstein's "Myth of the Noble Scientist," they often don't represent the true chronology of events or the intricacies of assembling and interpreting facts that have led to conclusions. Moreover, scientific papers rarely describe or put into perspective the pure luck and mistakes that were also part of the work being reported. Frederick Grinnell, discussing the writing of Medawar, describes the scientific paper's purpose as providing the necessary information and arguments for accepting a discovery (6). In short: "Other researchers will expect to be able to verify the data and the conclusions, not the adventures and misadventures that led to them."

Henry Bauer has written about what he terms the Myth of the Scientific Method (1). He contends that scientific research rarely proceeds by the organized, systematic approach that is reflected in textbook discussions of the scientific method. Approaches to solving problems and answering questions exhibit varying blends of empiricism and theorizing. Depending on the discipline as well as the intellect and personality of the scientist, research proceeds with considerable variations on the scientific method. Bauer argues that science varies immensely in its characteristics. On a broad scale, he proposes a set of categories which he terms "textbook science" and "frontier science." The former has withstood the scientific scrutiny of time and is not likely to be subject to frequent change. The latter is often termed "cutting-edge" science. It is volatile, sometimes unreliable, and subject to considerable change. Bauer correctly points out that textbook science fails to reveal the true workings of scientific exploration, as it teaches us only about successful science. Hence, it is not an accurate portrayal of the often convoluted pathway that leads to accepted and relatively stable scientific results. Such end products of research commonly are the result of multiple investigational efforts, representing different lines of intellectual and technological approach. Such efforts can occur over lengthy periods of time, in which corroborative and contradictory evidence must be addressed and, where necessary, reconciled. Textbook science evolves to a point of general acceptance with the caveat that future knowledge may further refine, modify, or even disprove it. To attempt to explain this process as the result of the systematic implementation of a single, prescribed scientific method sheds little light on the process of how science actually works.

Bauer's concept of frontier science in relation to scientific integrity is particularly relevant. This brand of science by definition invites examination and scrutiny. Methods, data, interpretations, and conclusions are called into question as part of this process. Herein emerge issues like "honest error" and differences in judgment. Unfortunately, the rigorous analysis of frontier science can lead to erroneous perceptions and misunderstanding that can translate to accusations of scientific misconduct. Scientists' intuition as applied to a problem and their personal judgments and decisions may be targeted and subjected to scrutiny in ways that can take on an air of investigation. Who is to say that a scientist's applying his or her intuition to a problem is a bad judgment or is sloppy science, as opposed to being done deliberately to deceive? Deciding to discount enzyme assay data that were obtained from protein preparations extracted from what a biochemist might call "unhealthy cells" serves as a hypothetical case in point. Can intuition be relied upon to recognize potentially flawed data? Such are the gray areas that scientists must think about and address both as practitioners and as critics. Clearly, scientific intuition can be applied in a way that allows the investigator to make a major conceptual advance. Robert Millikan's selective publication of data on the electric charges of oil drops led to an understanding of the particulate nature of electric charge (1,4). His intuition led him to discount data involving the migration of electrically charged oil drops which didn't conform to his expectations because they had "something wrong" with them. Millikan's work is clearly recognized in terms of what Bauer would call textbook science. Scientific integrity issues about Millikan's work have been raised in recent times, however (2,4). His intuition played an important role in his scientific achievement. However, the facts indicate that Millikan did not publish all of his data. Thus, at issue is not that Millikan discarded certain of the data gathered from some of the oil drops, but that in his published work on the subject he wrote that he presented all of his available data.

In fact, many have concluded that there is no single scientific method (1,8,11). Scientists use many different strategies and methods in their exploration of nature. Rarely, if at all, is the process ordered, even though scientific publications of frontier science present information in a way that bespeaks a logical and ordered progression of the research. Rather than a single, uniformly applied scientific method, there are many variations on this theme. Bauer submits that we view the classic description of the scientific method as an ideal rather than a specific formula for performing research. He further suggests that the projection of the concept of a prescribed scientific method provides society with unrealistic expectations of science and scientists. Scientists themselves are similarly misled.

Defining a universal scientific method against which we measure the integrity of the research process is neither practical nor logical. Howard Schachman's blunt assessment on prosecution of scientific misconduct carries this message: "...it is inappropriate, wasteful, and likely to be destructive to science for government agencies to delve into the styles of scientists and their behavioral patterns" (10). Goodstein (5) further argues that the codification of methods for defining, monitoring, and prosecuting scientific misconduct is dangerous "...because it assumes there is a single set of practices commonly accepted by the scientific community and [it] sets up a government agency to root out the deviations from those practices."

Conclusion

The practice of science has always encompassed values that include honesty, objectivity, and collegiality. The progress of science in the latter half of this century is but one fitting tribute to the success of the research enterprise. Clearly there is nothing fundamentally wrong with the conduct of science. However, emphasis on the workings of science and the conduct of scientists has shifted considerably in recent years.

Governmental oversight and definitions of scientific misconduct sometimes lead one to believe that scientific integrity is a new concept. However, scientific integrity existed long before definitions were written and promulgated, and there would be integrity in science even if definitions did not exist. The codes that govern conduct in science are likely to grow more explicit in years to come, as indicated in part by the recent focus on articulation of misconduct definitions. These are practical matters that cannot be ignored by scientists. Here, we have crystallized a number of issues related to scientific conduct to get both students and practitioners of science to think about them in both theoretical and practical ways.

REFERENCES

1. **Bauer, H.** 1992. *Scientific Literacy and the Myth of the Scientific Method.* University of Illinois Press, Chicago.
2. **Broad, W., and N. Wade.** 1982. *Betrayers of the Truth: Fraud and Deceit in the Halls of Science.* Simon and Schuster, New York.
3. **Buzzelli, D. E.** 1993. A definition of misconduct in science: a view from NSF. *Science* **259**:584–585, 647–648.
4. **Goodstein, D.** 1991. Scientific fraud. *Am. Scholar* **60**:505–515.
5. **Goodstein, D.** 1992. What do we mean when we use the term scientific fraud? *Scientist,* March 2, p. 11–13.
6. **Grinnell, F.** 1992. *The Scientific Attitude.* The Guilford Press, New York.
7. **Medawar, P. B.** 1981. *Advice to a Young Scientist.* Harper & Row, New York.
8. **Medawar, P. B.** 1984. *The Limits of Science.* Oxford University Press, Oxford.
9. **National Academy of Sciences.** 1992. *Responsible Science,* Vol. 1: *Ensuring the Integrity of the Research Process.* National Academy Press, Washington, D.C.
10. **Schachman, H. K.** 1993. What is misconduct in science? *Science* **261**:148–149, 183.
11. **Wolpert, L.** 1993. *The Unnatural Nature of Science.* Harvard University Press, Cambridge, MA.
12. **Zurer, P. S.** 1993. Ethical issues underlying responsible conduct of science explored. *Chem. Eng. News,* March 15, p. 7–10.

2 | *Mentoring*

Francis L. Macrina

Overview

In research training, a mentor is defined as someone who is ultimately responsible for the guidance and the academic, technical, and ethical development of a student. Mentoring extends well beyond the training phase of one's professional development and mentor–disciple or mentor–protegé relationships may continue throughout the better part of one's career, in science as well as in virtually all professional disciplines. This chapter primarily discusses predoctoral mentoring, referring to the participants as "mentor" and "trainee." Some of what will be said applies to mentoring of the postdoctoral trainee as well. Career mentoring at later professional stages involves many of the basic principles and strategies that are employed in mentoring trainees at the predoctoral level.

The canons of scientific integrity derive from effective mentoring in graduate training programs. Mentors inform, instruct, and provide an example for their trainees. The actions and activities of mentors affect the intellect and attitude of their trainees. The educational transfer process may be obvious or subtle, but the effects are rarely in dispute: trainees emerge from their programs with an intellectual and ethical framework strongly shaped by their mentors. Indeed, trainees often assume the traits and values of their mentors. Thus, mentors are the stewards of scientific integrity. Those who, by example, signal their trainees that productivity is more important than proper scientific conduct are neglecting their responsibilities. In examining cases of reported scientific misconduct, mentorship issues, duties, and responsibilities often are brought to the forefront of the discussion as being

15

central. Yet, the young faculty member who has just accepted his or her first trainee into the lab is not likely to have had much formal education in the principles of mentoring and is very likely to have no experience in it at all. The direct experience of dealing with trainees improves mentoring skills. To be sure, the skills and responsibilities of mentoring sometimes elude precise articulation and definition since, as a human-centered activity, there is naturally great variation in practice. There are many effective styles and, though common traits may be shared, there is no one prescribed method.

Characteristics of the Mentor–Trainee Relationship

In the graduate biomedical sciences at the predoctoral level, mentoring has several important characteristics. Perhaps most important, the mentor teaches and provides the intellectual support for the trainee. Mentors have been described variously by using words like advisor, advocate, critic, and instructor. Serving as a role model or scientific parent are two additional descriptions that illuminate the mentor's participation in the training experience.

Clarice Yentsch and C. J. Sindermann (13) prepared from personal interviews the following list of activities of mentors:

- Demonstrating a style and methodology of doing research
- Developing an analytical approach to selection of significant questions and choosing appropriate approaches to solving them
- Discussing the concepts in any subdiscipline, and the evolution of those concepts over time
- Exploring and evaluating the literature of the discipline and the broader body of knowledge of which it is a part
- Discussing the ethical basis for scientific research
- Considering, analyzing, and evaluating the work and conclusions of colleagues
- Transmitting, by example and discussions, the skills required for effective scientific writing
- Evaluating successful teaching techniques
- Facilitating access to the research community in the discipline (scientific societies, peer groups, international science, "in groups," etc.)

- Illustrating the methodology and significance of "networking" in science
- Developing attitudes and approaches to the many interpersonal relationships involved in being a scientist

Mentoring involves differing activities at different times. The primary duties of a mentor change over a time frame that varies enormously. Switching from discharging one's duties as mentor–advisor to mentor–confidant to mentor–critic might occur over the span of a day or even over a few hours. Changing one's mentoring demeanor as appropriate requires critical personal attention and oversight. Mentoring is a one-on-one activity. It is correctly depicted as an intense relationship between mentor and trainee that demands continued personal and intellectual involvement on the parts of both parties. Mentoring relationships are intricate interpersonal relationships that work best in an atmosphere of mutual respect, trust, and compassion. Mentoring is dynamic and complex. Simplifying the scope of mentoring duties and responsibilities is misleading and counterproductive. David Guston (3) correctly points out "what the mentor role is *not.*" A mentor is not just a patron (resource advisor), or just a supervisor (overseeing a dissertation), or an institutional linkage between student and the academic administration or, finally, just a role model. Mentoring roles overlap and receive differing emphases depending on specific circumstances and the changing needs of the trainee.

One of the unique aspects of predoctoral mentoring is the degree to which the trainee is dependent upon the mentor. In many cases, this dependence is grounded in finances, with the mentor's grant providing stipend support and often tuition and fee payments. Almost without exception in the biomedical sciences, the mentor's grant provides the resources which are critically needed for trainees to perform and complete their dissertation research. Moreover, the mentor is usually directly or indirectly involved in providing or securing the resources for trainees to attend meetings or workshops which are important to their graduate training experience. Finally, trainees are critically dependent on their mentors for a position when they finish their programs. Such positions might entail postdoctoral training, or employment in academics, industry, or government. This dependence on the evaluation of the mentor continues well into the trainee's career—applying for a position beyond a postdoctoral training experience usually involves the predoctoral mentor's providing a letter of recommendation on behalf of the trainee.

Thus graduate trainees are profoundly dependent on their mentors and similar dependencies are encountered in the postdoctoral trainee–mentor relationship. This dependence warrants discussion in terms of the vulnerability of the trainee to abuses of power. Although such abuse would seem antithetical to the basic premise of mentoring, trainees do fall victim to such circumstances. Abuses of power can take the form of acts of commission as well as acts of neglect. The trainee usually finds himself or herself in a difficult position when such situations emerge. The very person that should be available to solve the problem at hand turns out to be at the heart of the problem. Nonetheless, the mentor should be directly approached if such problems are being perceived by the trainee. Communication between mentor and trainee can be an effective way to resolve the situation. In addition, graduate advisory committees, other faculty, and departmental chairs can usually help in these circumstances. However, it is usually best to take up the issue with one's mentor first. Problems of this type progress to complicated proportions if the trainee fails to address them in a timely fashion. Because they are largely dependent upon their mentors at a time when they feel abused by the same person, trainees may find themselves facing a dilemma that is not easily resolved. Avoiding direct communication is a virtual guarantee that the problem will get worse.

The mentor–trainee relationship is a rather exclusive one. Although graduate programs usually mandate that each predoctoral trainee be guided by an advisory committee, the mentor chairs such a committee and is the trainee's principal advocate in this forum. At times, however, members of the graduate advisory committee or even other faculty may assume transient mentoring roles. For example, a trainee in biochemistry may need to produce antibodies against a protein she has isolated. To achieve this goal, she may be scientifically mentored by an immunologist who may or may not sit on her advisory committee. Mentoring activities in this case might involve instruction and advice regarding compliance with regulations concerning the use of animals in research, the handling of animals in the called-for experiments, and relevant immunological methods needed to do the work.

The largely exclusive and intense nature of the mentor–trainee association in science is underscored by the usual longevity of such relationships. Predoctoral mentoring in graduate biomedical research usually marks the beginning of a relationship that significantly outlives the actual time spent in formal training. Trainees often continue to rely on their graduate mentors for advice and counsel as they enter and progress through the beginning stages of their professional careers. Mentors are often viewed in the light of the performance of their former trainees and this can indefinitely extend the responsibilities of the relationship from the mentor's point of view. Carl Djerassi points out that evidence of the mentoring relationship can sometimes be found even after the mentor's death (2).

For a mentor to remain in touch with the academic status, intellectual development, and practical research progress of a trainee, regular oversight, information exchange, and frequent and regular interpersonal communication are required. This principle serves as a useful guide for assessing one's ability to function effectively as a mentor. One critical issue is that of research group population size. As the number of both predoctoral and postdoctoral trainees increases (not to mention increases in the numbers of technical staff) there simply becomes less time to conduct a proper and effective mentor–trainee relationship. Mentors need to face up to this reality as they weigh commitment, take on additional responsibilities, and, in general, "grow" their research training programs. There is a point of diminishing returns in terms of the number of trainees that can be effectively mentored. When that threshold is crossed, the ability to responsibly guide trainees is compromised and the viability of the training experience is put in jeopardy. Poorly mentored trainees can unknowingly cut corners, make mistakes, or not recognize errors. Over time, such behavior can come back to haunt mentors by jeopardizing the credibility of their research programs. Thus, neglect of mentoring responsibilities and duties can harm both mentors and trainees.

Certain fundamental characteristics must pervade the mentor–trainee relationship. Personal respect is absolutely necessary on both sides of the mentoring relationship; mentors have an obligation to respect and preserve the individual dignity of their trainees. Robert Audi (1) has looked at graduate training in this context.

> Students are never to be treated as a means—say, just an essential element in a successful academic career—but always as beings with a certain dignity. They are, by implication, to be treated with respect and, at times, their teach-

ers must become advocates for them, whether internally in relations with administrators or other faculty members or externally in helping them secure a position. The same applies, of course, to students' treatment of professors, who are not to be viewed as merely means to a degree or a career.

Mutual trust is another essential ingredient for a successful mentoring relationship. Throughout the relationship, the trainee must trust the mentor's advice and actions that bear on his or her training programs. Most students at the early stages of their programs depend strongly, if not exclusively, on their mentor's knowledge and expertise in helping select a viable dissertation research project. A mentor who has developed a reputation for recommending changes in a trainee's dissertation project at the least sign of failure may have difficulty attracting and keeping students in her or his lab. Such actions tend to reduce confidence and undermine trust in the mentor's scientific decisionmaking style. Mentors, on the other hand, cultivate a trust in the caliber of work performed by the trainee over the course of the dissertation research project. During an active mentoring relationship the mentor is able to gauge a trainee's performance by three principal means: (1) direct laboratory observation, (2) viewing the trainee's raw and analyzed research data, and (3) listening to trainees present their ideas and data in both informal and formal settings. Over time, the mentor develops a degree of confidence in the trainee's operating style based on these observations. Such observations continue throughout the course of graduate training to a greater or lesser degree. Direct laboratory observation usually is a significant component in the early stages of training, but may wane and even disappear as the trainee progresses and matures. Data observation and related discussion persists throughout the entire course of the trainee mentoring experience. This activity should be characterized by regular face-to-face meetings, with databooks and other relevant materials in hand. The mentor should observe trainees as they present seminars or research reports or participate in journal clubs. This activity should persist throughout the training experience and serves two functions. First, it allows for continuing evaluation of student progress in scientific thinking and analyses. Second, it provides an excellent forum for the mentor to comment on and critique the scientific communication skills of the trainee.

Free and open communication flows from an atmosphere of mutual respect and trust in a successful mentor–trainee relationship. Good mentors are critical and demanding of their trainees and these characteristics should be explicit in all forms of communication. Constructive criticism should prevail in such proceedings. When mixed with compassionate personal support and enthusiasm for the work, trainees are likely to recognize helpful criticism and guidance and not confuse these messages with displeasure, hostility, or intimidation. Such interchange, in turn, cultivates a collegial relationship between the participants as they share and analyze information, critique each other's ideas, and solve problems with each other's help. Attribution of credit and recognition of accomplishments should be clearly articulated in the ongoing dialogue. Taken together, these activities are the important first steps in the broad-based socialization of a young scientist. Indeed such mentoring activities are setting the stage for a career's work in science. That is, these same activities continue throughout a scientist's career in differing contexts and scales.

Mentor Selection

In their books on graduate research, authors Robert Smith (9) and Molly Stock (10) have written about the kinds of issues that students may wish to consider in selecting graduate advisors. Recognizing that most graduate students enter training programs and then choose a mentor sometime during their first year or so of study, these authors suggest a variety of both subjective and objective criteria that may be useful. Combining their suggestions yields the following list of issues a trainee may wish to consider in selection of a mentor.

- Active publication record in high-quality, peer-reviewed journals
- Extramural financial support base: competitiveness and continuity of support
- National recognition: meeting and seminar invitations, invited presentations, consultantships
- Rank, tenure status, and proximity to retirement age
- Prior training record (time to complete degree and numbers of graduates) and enthusiasm for previous trainee's accomplishments
- Current positions of recent graduates

- Recognition for student accomplishments (e.g., coauthorship practices)
- Laboratory organizational structure and direct observation of the laboratory in operation

Acquiring such information is possible but frequently requires that students have access to documents such as curriculum vitae and departmental records, such as annual reports. This kind of fact finding is undoubtedly useful for some prospective trainees. Mentoring experience tends to indicate that most students, for better or for worse, do not actively gather this kind of information in any organized or systematic way. It is rare that first year graduate students ask to inspect the curriculum vitae of a prospective mentor; neither are such students likely to seek out and read a copy of the most recent departmental annual report to check on grant funding status, publication record, etc. In fact, many trainees get varying amounts of this kind of information in conversations with potential mentors and their students; facts get transmitted both passively (not in response to any line of questioning) and in response to direct queries. Departmental advertising in the form of posters or brochures and descriptions of research programs also provide a baseline of information on potential mentors.

In practice, mentor selection usually centers around three principal activities. The first is education. The trainee can read research descriptions in advertising documents as well as published works of the prospective mentor to determine if his or her interests coincide with that of his or her graduate training goals. For the student who has entered graduate school with little thought as to areas of interest, this kind of analysis is not likely to provide much of a focus. On the other hand, consider a student who has entered into a graduate biochemistry program. Exposure to a variety of readings enables the student to explore training opportunities that might involve disparate areas within the chosen discipline. In biochemistry, this might include molecular genetic approaches to study enzyme catalysis in one lab, biochemistry of DNA replication in another lab, or X-ray crystallographic analysis of macromolecules in yet a third faculty laboratory.

The second important activity in mentor selection is interpersonal interaction, both with the potential mentor and with members of his or her research group. It is in the best interest of the potential mentor and trainee to meet on several occasions and to discuss thoroughly the practical issues of dissertation research possibilities and the logistics of selection of a project. It is also appropriate to cover issues such as mentoring style, including level of supervision, general expectations and goal setting, and other personal and academic issues related to graduate training. Candid discussion at this point not only provides the basis for an intelligent decision on the part of both prospective trainee and mentor but also sets the stage for the free and open communication that must support the trainee–mentor relationship during formal academic training and dissertation research. Talking with lab members about their view of the training environment provides a valuable perspective as well. Training climate, enthusiasm of other trainees, and corroborative information on the mentoring style of the laboratory head can make the potential trainee comfortable with the prospects for selecting a mentor, or can raise questions which will likely need to be answered by the prospective mentor.

A third useful activity in the mentor selection process stems from the existence of lab rotation programs now found in many graduate biomedical science departments. Such programs typically involve the first-year graduate student doing a specific research project (or learning specialized methodology) over the course of a few to several weeks. This provides a first-hand view of the operation of the lab and its personnel dynamics, including mentor–trainee relationships. This interaction is often a first exposure to the day-to-day perspective of a research environment for many entering graduate students. Such primary exposure allows prospective trainees to directly assess the climate they will encounter in their training experience. Does the mentor provide much direct supervision, or are technological skills and data analysis and interpretation relegated to another senior lab member? Has the training environment changed much over time in the experience of the trainee presently on board? Have the methods of training used by the mentor been successful? The rotation system also allows the mentor to view the prospective trainee at the research bench and, in doing so, acquire useful, albeit brief and casual, impressions of his or her potential.

In summary, mentor selection requires both formal and informal activities coupled with thoughtful analyses on the part of both participants. However, even the most thoughtful decisions, based on the careful collection of facts and data, can result in mentor–trainee relationships that "do not work." Conflicting personal styles that emerge over time, disenchantment with some general area of research, and evolving changes in aspects of mentoring responsibilities or discharge of duties can all cause a mentor–trainee relationship to deteriorate. When this happens, early resolution is the best course of action for all involved. Candid mentor–trainee discussion of problems may need to be augmented by third party "mediators" or "negotiators" (e.g., departmental chairs or graduate program directors). Intractable problems should be recognized and accepted; switching mentors in a predoctoral training program can and should be implemented to solve such problems. Prolonging problems by failing to face up to them often creates tension in the training environment and can unnecessarily lengthen the duration of the training program.

Models

Robert Smith has described three types of mentor (9). These examples may risk oversimplification, but a brief discussion of his thesis can illuminate the perspectives of both the trainee and the mentor. The collaborator type of mentor is described as representing the professionally youthful individual, usually an assistant professor. Smith characterizes such individuals as being concerned with achieving productivity consistent with initiating professional development. Such development is linked to gaining extramural support and to seeking professional rewards like advancement in faculty rank. These mentors are more likely to work alongside trainees and, due to light or only emerging administrative duties, simply have more time to devote to the mentor–trainee relationship. According to Smith, collaborative-type mentors focus on productivity, which may lead to trainee research project choices that are of relatively low risk, so as to enhance research productivity. Collaborative advisors clearly have a vested interest in their students' research results. In fact, it can be argued that this premise holds for all of the mentor types that Smith describes. Graduate research results are a critical driving force in a lab where predoctoral training occurs. Directly or indirectly, the research efforts of trainees are linked to productivity—trainees' data ultimately become the basis of publications. In the biomedical and natural sciences, this productivity is critical to the establishment or the continuation and strengthening of grant support. In the university setting, where most predoctoral training occurs, the lack of such a funding base provides a virtual impasse to graduate biomedical research. Such work is expensive and university funding is almost never available to pay for it.

Smith's second mentor model is termed the hands-off type. Smith characterizes this type of mentor as one who is at some mid-level of academic rank and achievement. This mentor might be expected to be less demanding in terms of research results due to his or her professional confidence level. Smith suggests that a possible pitfall associated with this type of mentorship supervision is that it can allow excessive time to complete research. On the other hand, such a mentor might allow trainees to attack problems of relatively higher risk and, accordingly, reward and significance. Smith's final mentor type is described as the senior scientist advisor. Although usually overburdened with commitments of differing types, this individual can provide a kind of high-quality attention to trainees, although such attention and advising may be unpredictable in its timing.

Whether or not an oversimplification, Smith's mentor models highlight a continuum of styles that realistically comprise the individual nature of mentor approaches to training. Obviously, many permutations of the three types of mentoring styles exist. For example, mentors who fit the senior scientist description may actually practice their mentoring skills as collaborator types. They may deliberately control and curtail their participation in other assignments in order to be able to devote considerable amounts of time to mentoring duties. They may in fact work in the lab themselves, side-by-side with trainees. Like collaborator types, they have a vested interest in the research data of their trainees, because such information will ultimately translate into the productivity that will allow their scholarly programs and grant support to flourish. The experience of senior scientist types may dictate that they assign a relatively low-risk, low-significance project to a trainee based on their knowledge of the trainee's experience or academic performance. In reality, mentors may use varying styles with different trainees, or they may change their style with the same trainee at differing points in the training program (e.g., from a collaborator style to a more hands-off style as the trainee progresses). In summary, Smith's mentor models are built on the central issues of quality and quantity of attention that a mentor provides to a trainee. This is a valid and important way to analyze mentor styles. Potential trainees should have a good feel for the style of mentoring that a potential advisor practices. This information can be gleaned using the various strategies discussed above: from the mentor, from lab members, and from a lab rotation experience.

In discussing the ethics of graduate teaching, Robert Audi also invokes behavioral models that span all varieties of graduate teaching experience (1). He summarizes his four models using mottos: (1) the didactic model—"Listen to me"; (2) the apprentice model—"Follow me"; (3) the collegial model—"Be my junior colleague"; and (4) the friendship model—"Be my friend." Predoctoral mentoring in the biomedical sciences usually is a blending of these styles, influenced by the trainee's abilities, stage of training, and personal philosophy of the mentor. Depending on timing and personalities, specific mentoring may be dominated by one of these styles. Senior-level graduate trainees who have finished all courses and comprehensive exams and are writing research publications based on their original findings are likely to experience the collegial model in their relationship with their mentor. Entry-level trainees are more likely to experience a combination of the didactic and apprentice models.

The friendship model warrants further discussion here in the context of graduate training. Audi cautions that this model presents a challenge to the responsible professor (mentor). He contends that socialization with students makes it difficult to assign grades fairly, to evaluate critically befriended students, and to recommend them objectively for professional opportunities (e.g., positions). Further, he argues that detachment must be maintained in the relationship between professor and student. Audi's points should be carefully considered. The mentor–trainee relationship in the predoctoral or postdoctoral setting must not be compromised by any type of personal bias that might result from friendship. Interestingly, mentors and trainees, especially at the late stages of training, often describe themselves as "friends." The very nature of graduate training in the biomedical sciences makes it difficult for bonds of friendship not to form over time. Frequent interaction, working toward common goals, sharing thoughts and ideas, and solving problems together can foster friendship. Friendship that evolves in this setting can be maintained in the context of mutual compassion and support. Will extensions of this relationship necessarily compromise it and introduce unhealthy bias in dealing with trainees? Arguments can be made in both directions in situations where, for example, mentors regularly socialize with trainees outside of the laboratory–classroom setting (e.g., sports teams, regular recreational activities). Any resulting bias that is taken back to the lab or classroom would depend on the fundamental philosophy and characteristics of the mentor. Finally, mentor–trainee relationships between members of the opposite sex can and do cross the threshold from supportive friendship to include romance. Romantic involvement with one's trainee is inappropriate and must be avoided. Institutions have discussed these kinds of issues and some have drafted relevant guidelines and regulations forbidding such relationships.

Mentoring Guidelines

A number of institutions have written guidelines for the responsible conduct of research (4, 6, 7, 11, 12). Some of these documents begin with a preamble that affirms the importance of mentoring in scientific training. Unique characteristics of mentoring include the complexities of modern scientific technologies, the existence of interdisciplinary, collaborative research, the provision of guidance and caution in interpreting possibly ambiguous data, and the need for advanced statistical analysis of data. A compilation and distillation of the common points covered by these documents follows.

- Specific assignment of trainees to faculty preceptors (mentors) must be made, with responsibility for the trainee residing unambiguously with the faculty member

Mentoring relationships in predoctoral training begin with the assignment of a temporary advisor and continue throughout training with the selection of a dissertation advisor. The duties of the temporary advisor and the permanent advisor should be clearly articulated (preferably in writing).

- The ratio of mentor to trainees in a given laboratory should be small enough to foster scientific interchange and to afford supervision of the research activities throughout the training program

Few will argue with the assertion that at some point, the size of a laboratory research group may curtail or even preclude responsible and effective mentoring. However, defining that point is difficult, as it depends on a variety of factors including the type (entry level–

advanced, predoctoral–postdoctoral) of trainee, the nature of the work being performed, the overall commitments of the mentor's time, and the mentor's management skills. Most would argue that active mentoring of more than 10 to 12 trainees is not possible. Larger groups must have a "secondary mentoring" network in place, where senior members of the lab serve as mentors to trainees. Such an infrastructure may enable the laboratory head to delegate monitoring duties, but this practice is arguably not in keeping with mentoring guidelines as forwarded by some institutions. Specifically, mentoring is predicated on mentor–trainee interchange and, as such, does not typically afford the latitude for delegation of such responsibility.

- There should be a direct role for the mentor in supervising the design of experiments and all activities related to data collection, analysis and interpretation, and storage

The emphasis here is on close supervision of trainee's progress, highlighted by personal interaction. Some standards of conduct underscore the importance of direct, active supervision by providing a contrasting statement: "A preceptor who limits his / her role to the editing of manuscripts does not provide adequate supervision."

- Collegial discussion among mentors and trainees should pervade the relationship and should be highlighted by regular group meetings which contribute to scientific efforts of the group and, at the same time, expose trainees to informal peer review

In fact, regular group meetings should be augmented by mentor–trainee meetings that are held regularly and privately. Such individualized attention provides the mentor and trainee with an excellent opportunity for uninhibited communication, critical analysis, and problem solving that may be unique to the trainee or the specific project.

- The mentor is responsible for providing trainees with all relevant rules, regulations and guidelines that may apply to the conduct of research (e.g., documents concerning human and animal use or use of radioactive and hazardous substances)

The mentor has a responsibility for oversight and enforcement in this area too. Trainees must comply with rules and regulations as either observed directly or monitored indirectly by the mentor. Breach of any established policy will ultimately rest with the mentor as the individual with overall responsibility for the laboratory group.

In addition, one document lists some behavioral assessment-type issues which fall under the category of mentoring responsibilities. These include the formulation of "realistic expectations" for trainees' performance and their communication to the trainees. Mentors then have an obligation to provide a realistic appraisal of a trainee's performance. That document also advises mentors to be alert to behavioral changes in trainees which may be caused by stress or substance abuse. It specifically cites stresses due to transitions and deadlines and cautions that increased supervision may be needed at such times. Another institutional guideline emphasizes that the research laboratory experience should be at all times a learning experience, engendering appreciation of proper methods and conduct and appropriate ethical consideration of all those affected by the research. Finally, another document specifically defines the duty of a mentor to provide a meaningful training experience for a trainee. This is followed by the admonition that projects in which the mentor has a monetary or "compelling interest" are not acceptable training experiences.

A word about expectations for predoctoral trainees is in order. Early career mentors often rely on the departmental or graduate program guidelines to help them formulate trainee expectations. Seasoned mentors can benefit from using such documents as well. The language therein can be translated into easily understandable goals. When wedded to some time frame, such guidelines create a perspective that affords clear milestones for evaluation by the mentor while at the same time providing motivation for the trainee. Although this aspect of mentoring is general and rather pragmatic, it provides the foundation for communication and correctly transmits, from an early point, the active involvement of the mentor in the training process. As an extension of this manner of thinking, the International Union of Immunological Societies (IUIS) has recognized a need for uniform standards in graduate training in immunobiology. A proposal describing such guidelines has been published and serves as a useful model for discussion (8). This and similar documents (5) can help guide the clear articulation of expectations and standards to trainees. Ultimately, this can greatly assist the early evaluative steps of the training program.

Although timing for achievement of specific outcomes may vary based on experience and individual preference, the general standards of a given program might parallel those recommended by the IUIS report. These are presented and briefly annotated here to provide a useful example. They may be adapted to other disciplines.

- The candidate should demonstrate a general knowledge of basic immunology
  This means understanding experimental methods in a way that facilitates appreciation of basic concepts rather than merely accepting conclusions reached by others. It also implies requisite reading and comprehension of the primary and secondary scientific literature in the discipline. In the case of the IUIS report, specific examples of appropriate journals are listed. Mentors and graduate advisory committees should likewise offer guidance in journal reading to the new trainee. The candidate's level of understanding can be evaluated by direct observation by the mentor as well as by course work and comprehensive examination performance.
- The candidate should be familiar with the immunology literature and be able to acquire a working background knowledge of any area related to immunology
  The ability to read critically and to use such information to ask further questions and propose relevant research problems is essential. Active journal clubs (where students present and discuss the primary literature), seminars, research proposals, and research paper writing all provide good indicators of students' appreciation and comprehension of the literature.
- The candidate should possess technical skill
  Through course work or independent training and study the student must display the ability to master techniques needed to conduct the assigned dissertation research project. Evaluation in courses as well as the direct observation of laboratory techniques and resulting data is needed to assess performance.
- The candidate should ask meaningful questions
  Subjective evaluation by the mentor as well as reviewing the student's ability to critically evaluate the literature as a component of seminar presentations and writings provides an indication of performance. The IUIS report (8) points out that

"[a]cquisition of the ability to formulate meaningful questions is a major step in the candidate's transition from a passive to an active role in research."
- The candidate should demonstrate oral and written communication skills
  Seminar and journal club presentations are expected; regular participation may be specifically defined. Verbal communication skills are best honed through regular practice. Informal or, if appropriate, formal evaluation of performance should be provided by the mentor, graduate advisory committee, and other faculty. Comments and guidance should be constructive, candid, and provided at every opportunity. Writing skills are also improved through practice—informal peer review involving mentors, faculty, and scientific colleagues is essential.
- The candidate should demonstrate skill in designing experimental protocols and in conducting productive independent research
  These skills are evaluated by the mentor on a frequent basis and by the student's graduate advisory committee on a periodic basis. With time, evidence of progress in this area becomes apparent to the mentor as less description and detail are needed to launch the student into specific aspects of the project.
- The candidates and supervisor should adhere to the ethical rules accepted by the scientific community
  This point embraces the expectation that the mentor–trainee relationship is the principal vehicle for the scientific and professional socialization of the trainee. It further expects that students will have available to them appropriate relevant training opportunities (e.g., good laboratory practice, appropriate use of animals and human subjects).

In summary, careful articulation of expectations is essential to effective graduate training. They provide a perspective for the trainee and can serve to motivate her or him. Equally important, they help mentors in carrying out their duties by holding students to explicit, recognized standards which are easily communicated, are readily monitored, and can be reasonably enforced. They are of particular help to inexperienced mentors in providing them with specific parameters for guidance and evaluation. They can and should be worded in general terms, taking into account the variances of differing programs and disciplines while at the same time not inhibiting the creative processes that underlie graduate dissertation research.

Conclusion

Mentor–trainee relationships in science are critical to both the technical training and the professional socialization of young scientists. The selection process should involve an informed decision on the part of both participants, and the resulting relationship must be built on mutual trust and respect. It is a dynamic interpersonal relationship, with both parties having distinct responsibilities. Formalizing the responsibilities of mentors has occurred at some institutions where written documents provide guidance. Guidance on the responsibilities of trainees can often be found in departmental documents such as graduate program policies and in the writings of scholarly societies, as illustrated by the examples provided in this chapter.

Case Studies

2.1 A professor is approached by a graduate student from another department at her institution and asked to write a letter of recommendation for the student who is being considered for a postdoctoral position in the laboratory of Dr. Morgan at Research University. The professor declines to write a letter for the student, stating conflict of interest on the grounds that one of her own trainees is applying for a postdoctoral position in the same laboratory at the same institution. Comment on the appropriateness of the professor's decision regarding this situation.

2.2 Two research associates are engaged in a discussion over the responsibilities of mentors of research training laboratories. The discussion centers on a specific case in which one of the research associates has determined that her mentor is totally incapable of operating an ELISA reader. Although this instrument is used commonly in his research laboratory and the mentor routinely critiques data of his trainees obtained on the instrument, the research associate claims her mentor doesn't even know how to turn on the instrument. What sorts of responsibilities do mentors have with respect to instrument theory and operation in their discipline?

2.3 A graduate student is in the process of interviewing faculty as potential dissertation advisors. The student becomes intensely interested in one faculty member's research program and they have several lengthy discussions about potential projects that the student could pursue as part of his dissertation research. Late in these discussions, the student asks questions about the financial support of various projects. Specifically, the student insists on knowing the source and duration of the support, and the investigator's plans for continuing sustained support. The faculty member is put off by these questions, indicates that these are inappropriate concerns for the student, and refuses to provide the information. Are these appropriate questions for the student to ask? Is the faculty member's response justified?

2.4 A faculty mentor in an academic research laboratory containing several predoctoral and postdoctoral trainees frequently receives letters announcing junior-level positions for scientists in academics, industry, or government. He deals with these letters in a variety of ways. Sometimes he posts them directly on the departmental bulletin board or on a bulletin board in his own laboratory. Other times he distributes them by using a routing list to faculty or to postdoctorals in the department. On occasion, he directly gives a letter to a postdoctoral trainee. Drs. Smith and Jones are currently postdoctoral trainees in this mentor's lab. Dr. Jones discovers Dr. Smith applying for a job at a prestigious university. In subsequent conversation, Dr. Smith freely discloses to Dr. Jones that the mentor provided him with a preadvertisement letter inviting applicants to apply for the position. Dr. Jones confronts the mentor and indicates she is upset that she was not notified about this position. The lab mentor asserts that his policy is to deal with such letters selectively. He states that he could not support Dr. Jones for the position in question. Consequently he did not provide Dr. Jones with the letter in advance of the published advertisement. Comment on this situation, specifically discussing the mentor's policies. What are the mentor's responsibilities in such matters? If you were a postdoctoral trainee in the laboratory, what would be your expectations regarding such matters? As a mentor, what would your policy on such matters be? Why? How, if at all, would such a policy be communicated to your trainees?

2.5 A faculty member and potential trainee have met several times to discuss possible projects the student might work on as a doctoral dissertation. The faculty member concludes the last discussion by listing a series of rules that he applies uniformly to his trainees. He indicates that he wants the student to know the rules of his laboratory fully before making a decision to join the lab. Most of the issues covered are straightforward, reasonable, and come as no surprise to the student. However, one rule that the faculty member states concerns the student. Specifically, the faculty member says that he does not permit his trainees to enter into romantic relationships with one another. Should such a relationship develop, he insists that one of the members of the relationship find a new advisor and a new laboratory. The student argues immediately that this is direct interference with personal matters and that such relationships are of no concern to the advisor. The faculty members counters with the fact that twice in the past five years his laboratory has been significantly disrupted by romantic relationships between trainees. These situations have resulted in ill will, diminished productivity, and a negative effect on the overall morale of his laboratory group. The faculty member indicates that he has carefully considered the implications of such relationships and has decided that the only reasonable thing to do is to prevent the problems they create by asking those involved to decide which of the two of them will leave the laboratory. Discuss the issues of mentorship responsibilities, ethics, and conflict of interest which you feel are important to this situation.

2.6 A graduate student who is well into his research program is seen less and less during the day by his mentor and other members of the laboratory. It becomes apparent to the faculty advisor that the student is working very long hours evenings and nights at times when most of the other laboratory workers are not there. This persists for several weeks. Finally, the mentor approaches the student and requests that he spend more time during "standard working hours" in the lab. The mentor argues that interaction with her and with other members of the laboratory is important and that it is best for all involved to share intellectual interaction in the laboratory. The student argues that he can work much more efficiently with fewer people around. The student specifically cites the fact that a piece of equipment he was using in his research was continually busy throughout the daytime hours and prevented his performing needed experiments in a timely fashion. Indeed, the student argues that this was the "straw that broke the camel's back," forcing him into working unconventional hours. Both the faculty advisor and the student hold tight to their arguments and over the next several days the situation between them grows tense. Comment on this situation and consider what avenues might be pursued in order to bring about resolution of this conflict.

2.7 A second-year graduate student is mapping specific mutations in bacteria. She can gain critical data on the location of a single mutation by doing four separate genetic crosses. Such a battery of crosses to map a single mutation can be done in three days. The student feels she can easily map two mutations per week. She has a total of 12 mutants to map for this part of her dissertation research. She meets with her mentor, who strongly recommends that the student conduct her work so as to map no more than one mutation per week. The mentor explains that this is the student's first exposure to genetic mapping and each experiment should be allotted considerable time for data analysis and interpretation. The student is upset with her mentor's recommendation. She argues that such a plan will unfairly delay her. Comment on the appropriateness of the mentor's suggestion and the student's response.

2.8 A mid-level graduate student in the midst of a well-defined research program clones by using recombinant DNA techniques a gene from a bacterium which encodes a membrane protein. Although the discovery of this gene was unexpected, the student and his mentor agree that further characterization is warranted. The mentor indicates that the nucleotide sequence of the gene should be determined and the student agrees with this assessment. The mentor informs the student that she wants the nucleotide sequence to be determined by a commercial laboratory which does such analyses on a fee-for-service basis. The student argues that he has had no experience in determining DNA sequences and would like to learn the technology. The mentor comments that this would be time-consuming and would unnecessarily delay the student's progress in other areas. The mentor indicates that if the student is interested in learning DNA sequencing, he should enroll in a techniques course at a later time. The student is not receptive to this suggestion. Can the mentor's decision be justified in your view? Can you suggest resolutions to this problem?

2.9 A graduate student prepares a research proposal in the form of an NIH grant application as part of her requirements for the Ph.D. degree. The idea for the proposal was generated by the student after reading a funded grant application of her mentor. However, the student has developed the idea thoroughly and the mentor has provided minimal assistance in the synthesis of the student's grant proposal. Several months later, the student learns that verbatim sections of her grant proposal have been included in a new grant application being submitted to NIH by her mentor. Comment on the appropriateness of the mentor's use of the student's written material. The student wishes to confront her mentor over this issue and has come to you for advice. What advice do you give her?

2.10 A postdoctoral fellow who has been associated with a large research group for three years has accepted a job at a university and is in the last few months of his formal training. His mentor asks to meet with him privately about a month before his departure from the laboratory and produces a typewritten document that summarizes the postdoctoral's contributions during his training. Moreover, the mentor specifically lists biological materials that the postdoctoral will not be allowed to remove from the laboratory. Finally, the document spells out several areas not yet under investigation in the mentor's laboratory which the postdoctoral is forbidden to work on in his new position. There is a signature line for the postdoctoral at the end of the document indicating his agreement to its language. The mentor asks the postdoctoral to take the document home, read it carefully, and return it to him signed in the morning. The postdoctoral leaves the office and is quite upset with the mentor's action. He believes his mentor is acting selfishly and unethically. He comes to you seeking your advice and your feelings on this matter. What do you tell him?

2.11 A faculty member has received a large grant from an industrial source to perform basic research that has long-term implications for commercialization. A new graduate student trainee has just joined his lab following the completion of one semester of graduate coursework. The faculty member outlines several projects that can be pursued by the student under this industrially sponsored research program. He indicates that there is a proviso listed in the industrial grant agreement which says that all material to be submitted for publication first be reviewed (within 120 days) by the company. The faculty member points out that this presents only a minimal disruption to the normal publication process as compared with the unrestricted publication of material gathered under federal research grants. He also mentions that the positive aspects of working on this proposal include the fact that there is money in the grant for the student to travel to at least two meetings per year. Also the grant application provides money for the student to purchase a personal computer for his lab station while he is working on the project. Finally, the faculty member emphasizes that working on the project will likely give the student an "inside track" with the company should he want to pursue job possibilities there following graduation. The student agrees to work on the project sponsored by the industrial grant. Comment on the ethical and conflict of interest implications of this scenario.

2.12 A faculty member is the graduate advisor for several predoctoral students. One of the students reports data to her advisor which describe a novel property of an enzyme under study. Both the advisor and the graduate student agree that this work has major implications for expanding knowledge around this enzyme. The student repeats her experiments and presents her advisor with data that are very similar to her previous results. Her advisor suggests that she do the experiments one more time to ensure reproducibility. Because of the important implications of this work, the advisor approaches another predoctoral student in the lab and asks the student to perform the same experiments in order to double-check the results. She instructs the student to perform the experiments without discussing them with anyone else in the lab in order to provide independent data to confirm these potentially important findings. Are the advisor's actions justified in this case? Why or why not?

2.13 A major portion of a student's doctoral dissertation is being prepared as a manuscript for submission to a peer-reviewed journal. The first draft of the manuscript prepared by the student has been heavily edited by the mentor. The mentor has even suggested some additional experiments for the student to do, including the suggestion that the two recombinant proteins under study be analyzed by circular dichroism (CD). She suggests that this be done collaboratively with a biophysical chemist in another department. Both the mentor and the student agree that this would be a significant contribution and would add considerable strength to the paper. The collaboration is set up over the course of the following two weeks. The mentor then tells the student that she would like him to audit a graduate level course in biophysical techniques being offered in the next semester. The mentor feels strongly that the student should have reasonable command of CD techniques if the student's paper is going to contain CD data. The student is within one year of completing all of his degree requirements. He strongly objects to the mentor's suggestion, stating that he can gain the necessary working knowledge to defend the collaboratively obtained CD data by reading on his own. Comment on this situation. What are the responsibilities of the student and the mentor in the collaborative arrangement? What, if any, are the responsibilities of the biophysical chemist who will do the CD studies? Are there other alternatives you can suggest in this situation?

REFERENCES

1. **Audi, R.** 1990. The ethics of graduate teaching, p. 119–149. *In* S. M. Cahn (ed.), *Morality, Responsibility, and the University—Studies in Academic Ethics.* Temple University Press, Philadelphia.
2. **Djerassi, C.** 1991. Mentoring: a cure for science bashing? *Chem. Eng. News,* November 25, p. 30–33.
3. **Guston, D.** 1993. Mentorship and the research training experience, p. 50–65. *In Responsible Science—Ensuring the Integrity of the Research Process,* Vol. II. National Academy Press, Washington, D.C.
4. **Harvard University Faculty of Medicine.** 1992. *Faculty Policies on Integrity in Science.* Boston.
5. **International Union of Biochemistry, Committee on Education.** 1989. Standards for the Ph.D. degree in biochemistry and molecular biology. *Trends Biochem. Sci.* **14:**205–209.
6. **The Johns Hopkins University School of Medicine.** 1990. *Faculty Policies.* Baltimore.
7. **National Institutes of Health.** 1990. *Guidelines for the Conduct of Research at the National Institutes of Health.* Bethesda, MD.
8. **Revillard, J.-P., and F. Celada.** 1992. Guidelines for the Ph.D. degree in immunology. *Immunol. Today* **13:**367–373.
9. **Smith, R. V.** 1990. *Graduate Research—A Guide for Students in the Sciences,* p. 23–42. Plenum Press, New York.
10. **Stock, M.** 1985. *A Practical Guide to Graduate Research,* p. 8–32. McGraw-Hill, New York.
11. **University of Michigan Medical School.** 1989. *Guidelines for the Responsible Conduct of Research.* Ann Arbor, MI.
12. **University of Minnesota.** 1989. *Guidelines for Research Investigators and Creative Artists.* Minneapolis, MN.
13. **Yentsch, C., and C. J. Sindermann.** 1992. *The Woman Scientist—Meeting the Challenge for a Successful Career,* p. 145–159. Plenum Press, New York.

3 | Scientific Record Keeping

Francis L. Macrina

Introduction

Proper record keeping is crucial to scientific research. However, accepted practices of record keeping and policies on custody and retention of data are subjects that are learned passively by many scientists. Informal surveys often reveal that trainees have received little instruction in the principles of scientific record keeping. When mentors don't communicate their expectations on the subject, trainees learn the practice of record keeping by trial and error and by having mentors correct their "mistakes." Some scientific misconduct investigations have reinforced the importance of keeping proper laboratory records (4). The creation of federal, institutional, or other professional standards for writing and maintaining laboratory databooks has even been suggested. Few, if any, granting agencies provide guidance on keeping laboratory records. Although contract-type research awards often define record keeping requirements, most of the funds that support graduate training in the biomedical sciences fail to provide any sort of a mandate for record keeping associated with graduate thesis or dissertation research.

Discussions of scientific record keeping run the risk of implying some uniform prescription for the process—a rigid method for the correct way to do things. However, like the resolution of the case studies in this text, there are multiple right ways to keep scientific records. So, although this chapter will have much to say about keeping a laboratory databook, its message is not an exact prescription or set of immutable rules. The nature of the research, the form and amount of data generated, and the preferences and practical experiences of individual scientists all affect the process. There are many styles and permutations that are proper and effective. Conversely, there are also practices that are improper or even scientifically irresponsible. This chapter has been written from the perspective of the academic or research institution laboratory setting. It considers issues and responsibilities related to doing sponsored research either as an independently funded investigator or a scientist-trainee.

Howard Kanare's text *Writing the Laboratory Notebook* is a definitive work on this subject (3). Its technical and detailed style is informative and useful. The Kanare text serves trainees and scientists well in thoroughly covering the key elements of laboratory record keeping. The book is worth owning and reading; this chapter draws heavily from its teachings.

Why Do We Keep Records?

Kanare defines and describes the laboratory databook as "...a bound collection of serially numbered pages used to record the progress of scientific investigations.... It contains a written record of the researcher's mental and physical activities from experiment and observation, to the ultimate understanding of physical phenomena." Keeping in mind a facile definition of the databook such as this is an important first step toward good scientific record keeping. Such records provide the platform for analysis and interpretation of results obtained in the field or the laboratory. They are the basis for scholarly writings including reports, grant and patent applications, journal articles, and theses and dissertations. Laboratory databooks are the definitive source of facts and details. Good record keeping fosters the scientific norms of accuracy, replication, and reliability. Corroboration and verification of scientific results using primary data contained in a laboratory databook may involve individuals other than the primary databook keeper. A scientist or scientist-trainee may take over a project and it would be necessary for him or her to understand precisely the laboratory databook contents in order to continue the work. Thus, a specific databook may become a key research tool for someone else in the laboratory group, or even someone outside the laboratory or the institution. This makes clarity and completeness of the laboratory databook essential to its usefulness.

Proper databook keeping also has legal implications and responsibilities. First, many agencies which fund biomedical science expect that good research records will be kept. For example, the National Institutes of Health (NIH) has the legal right to audit and examine records which are relevant to any research grant award. It follows that recipients of research grants have an obligation to keep appropriate records of experimental activities even though granting agencies such as NIH rarely provide guidance on how to do this. Second, the provision of primary research data is often a component of the approval process for new drugs or medical applications (e.g., data submitted to the U.S. Food and Drug Administration). For this type of activity, requirements for record keeping can be explicit. Failure to conform to such specifications can compromise the validity of the data and the utility of the research. Finally, scientific record keeping is a critical element in proprietary issues. As one seeks the protection of intellectual property by applying for a patent (see Chapter 8), it may become necessary to disclose databook contents to the patent examiner. Such disclosure might be related to requests for additional supporting data, dates of experiments or discoveries, verification that the records had been properly witnessed, or proof of reduction to practice. Properly kept databooks continue to be important after a patent is issued. Patents can be legally challenged once they are in force. Litigation involving such challenges may require that original databooks be inspected as part of the legal proceedings. Patents in whole or in part can be nullified as the result of such legal activities. A well-kept databook is an important factor in strengthening the claims allowed in the issued patent.

Defining Data

What do we mean by data? Simply stated, data are any form of factual information used for reasoning. Scientific data are not limited to the contents of databooks. Much of what we would call data contained in databooks is commonly classified as being intangible. That is, it contains handscript or affixed typescript which records and reports measurements, observations, calculations, interpretations, and conclusions. The term "tangible data," on the other hand, is used to describe materials such as cells, tissues or tissue sections, biological specimens, gels, photographs and micrographs, and other physical manifestations of research.

Data are said to have authenticity and integrity. Authentic data represent the true results of work and observations. When data deviate from this standard because of carelessness, self-deception, or deliberate misrepresentation, they lose their authenticity. Integrity of data is dependent on results being collected using well-chosen scientific methods carried out in the proper manner.

During the course of experimentation, some kinds of data evolve into different forms. Let's say you set out to do an electrophoretic analysis of some proteins. Your experiment results in a polyacrylamide gel in which a mixture of several proteins has been electrophoretically separated in a single lane. Also present in another lane of the gel are a series of reference proteins of known molecular weight and concentration. You visualize the protein components by staining with Coomassie blue dye. Then you desiccate the gel and seal it in a clear plastic envelope. You photograph the gel and the resulting print and negative are placed in plastic sleeves and taped into your databook; the desiccated gel is also taped to a databook page. Next, you calculate the apparent molecular weights of the proteins by comparing their migration relative to the standards. You do this by making measurements on both the gel and the photograph. In both of these cases, the data become transformed into handwriting in the databook. Then you enter your measurements into a computer which generates a numerical data set which is fixed as a printed copy; it is also maintained as an electronic file. You use a computer algorithm to determine the apparent molecular weights and you compare the results obtained by the different methods. Can you ascribe value to the various forms of the data which have come from this work? Is the gel itself the most important piece of data? Or, could the gel be discarded once it is recorded photographically? This scenario can be made more complex. For example, you scan the photographic negative using a digital scanner, resulting in its image being captured in an electronic file which is then printed on plotter paper. You use these electronic data to quantitate the proteins by comparing them to the concentrations of the proteins present in a control lane on the gel. You also use these data to make measurements electronically, enabling the program to compute the molecular sizes of the proteins.

It follows that all forms of data being considered—desiccated gel, photographic, electronic, and written or printed formats—are legitimate. Electronic technologies are changing how data are acquired, handled, and stored. The questions of identifying legitimate data strongly affect data analysis. Some forms of data may be better used for measurements and calculations than others. In the example given, it can be argued that measurements made from an optically or electronically generated image are more uniform from experiment to experiment as opposed to those taken directly from the gel. Other parts of this example raise issues about data storage. Is it better to emphasize the long-term storage of desiccated gels or to rely exclusively on a photographic or electronically derived image?

Terms like "raw data," "original data," and "primary data" are often used by scientists, but their definitions are elusive and their use can be confusing. The changing face of data collection, now strongly affected by electronic technology, requires careful consideration of what constitutes legitimate and valid data. Relevant discussions are needed at the laboratory, institution, and granting agency levels. Thus far, definitions of scientific data have been of limited scope and usefulness. In general, institutions and granting agencies have done little to illuminate these issues. Yet, the definition of data is central to scientific integrity. Many issues surrounding scientific data need to be discussed by institutions and funding agencies. Science and scientists will be well served when the importance of multiple data forms has been clarified and defined. Knowledge about data custody and storage, data removal and duplication, and disposal of data must lead to clear definitions and, where needed, guidelines or policies.

Data Ownership

Chapter 8 deals extensively with data ownership, but a brief discussion of this topic is in order here. The details of data ownership usually are not considered by researchers when they are writing grant applications. Such issues aren't likely to be foremost in the minds of principal investigators the day the grant award letter appears in the mail. However, it is a fact that most funding agencies are clear on the issue of data ownership when it comes to sponsored research. As the primary and largest funding agency for biomedical research in the United States, NIH under the aegis of the U.S. Public Health Service (USPHS) provides guidance on data ownership related to work supported by its research grants. As a matter of both policy and practice, the USPHS recognizes the grantee institution as the owner of the data generated by NIH-funded research (5). NIH grants are made to institutions, not to individuals. The individual who submits the grant on behalf of the institution is called the principal investigator. In practice, the principal investigator is the steward of the federal funds and of all aspects of the research that is sponsored by that support. The principal investigator assumes the primary responsibilities for data collection, recording, storage, retention, and disposal. Grantee institutions (e.g., universities) usually operate so as to give maximum latitude and discretion to principal investigators. However, the discharge of these duties does not impinge upon, nor should it cloud, the issue of data ownership. For example, if the principal investigator resigns his or her position to take another one at a different university, the grant award, the equipment purchased from the grant funds, and all of the data are required to remain at the institution that initially received the award. However, permission is usually sought to transfer the grant award, some or all of the equipment, and the data to the principal investigator's new institution. The process to do this is formal and requires mutual consent of the involved parties: the granting agency, the current grantee institution, and the proposed grantee institution. If for some reason an agreement is not reached, the initial grantee institution can keep the award, assuming it has identified a new principal investigator who is acceptable to the granting agency. The principal investigator as an individual never legally has ownership of data. The transfer of data ownership, when it occurs, is between grantee institutions.

Grantee institutions impose few restrictions on how principal investigators exercise their responsibilities as stewards of federal grant awards. Principal investigators usually have full control over the data. Although ownership versus control of the data are quite separate issues in this context, they become blurred with respect to one another. The behavior of principal investigators varies greatly when it comes to policies of scientific record keeping. Dr. Smith may have no expectation or policies about the keeping of a databook. People in his lab may rely on common sense or the advice of more experienced colleagues or may educate themselves independently by reading in the subject. When even fundamental expectations about scientific record keeping are not communicated, there is little hope for appreciation of the related deeper issues. Dr. Smith's lab team members probably don't think about the databook contents as property, nor are they likely to consider matters of data custody, retention, duplication, or security. Dr. Jones, on the other hand, may instruct all members of her research team that data shall be recorded in bound databooks, according to specifications which she describes. She further instructs members of her research team that databooks always remain in the laboratory and that photocopies of the databooks be submitted to her for safekeeping on a weekly basis. She distributes written policies stating that databooks never leave the lab and that their contents are the property of the institution. Dr. Jones also makes clear that trainees or staff who leave the institution upon completion of their work must never remove original data or databooks. The examples of Drs. Smith and Jones stand in striking contrast. Principal investigators need to comply with the policies (explicit or implicit) of federal and other research funding agencies. Thus, despite the contrast with Dr. Smith's lab, Dr. Jones' practices should not be considered extreme. Leaving the practice of laboratory record keeping to chance is irresponsible.

In summary, neither the principal investigator nor any member of the laboratory research team owns the data generated under an NIH research grant. Informing trainees and staff about practical issues of record keeping is the responsibility of the principal investigator.

Data Storage and Retention

Requirements for the amount of time research data must be retained may vary for various public and private funding agencies. Principal investigators are obliged to know about the varying data retention requirements imposed by the agencies that fund their work. The NIH, for example, requires that data obtained under the aegis of an NIH grant be retained for 3 years beyond the date of the financial expenditure report. In contrast, original data supporting patents should be retained for 23 years beyond the issue date of the patent (3). Keeping such records is necessary in the event that a patent is legally challenged or disputed. Yet another example is the 10-year period imposed by the U.S. Food and Drug Administration for original results of nonclinical research studies.

It would be impractical, if not impossible, for a major research university to organize, implement, and maintain a uniform data storage system for all of its research projects. Logistical problems at most universities and research institutions places the responsibility for the storage of data squarely with the principal investigator. Therefore, it is essential that investigators have a clear understanding of the policies governing data ownership issues and data retention.

Tools of the Trade

Keeping original results and observations for significant periods of time requires the selection of appropriate materials for recording and storing data. An entire chapter of the Kanare book (3) is devoted to "The Hardware of Notekeeping." It includes appendices containing information on the suppliers of laboratory notebooks, adhesives for attaching material to databook pages, pens and inks, and even test kits for evaluating the content of databook paper.

Paper

Kanare's discussions on the quality of databook paper are thorough and technical and may be summarized as follows. Desirable paper for laboratory record keeping should be acid-free and buffered. Acidity resulting from the degradation of components such as starch and alum-rosin is a major deterrent to the permanence of paper. Lignins present in ground wood used to make some papers also are degraded, resulting in increased acidity. One hundred percent chemically purified wood (not mechanically ground) which is buffered with calcium carbonate provides the greatest stability and is recognized as being "permanent." Interestingly, papers containing rag content may be erroneously assumed to provide permanence, but sufficient impurities may be present which promote cellulose degradation and thus increase acidity. Increased rag content is correctly associated with durability (folding qualities and strength), but similar results may be found in papers made from long, purified wood fibers. Selection of databooks composed of paper which is considered permanent can be aided by consulting databook suppliers or manufacturers. Sometimes details of paper composition and preparation are printed on the notebook cover. The longevity of all laboratory databooks, however, is facilitated by proper storage. Strong light sources, especially sunlight, high humidity, extremes in temperature, and excessive dust can have undesirable effects on stored laboratory records.

Ink and pen type

Kanare makes recommendations on pens and ink to be used in record keeping. Graphite pencil is unacceptable on several grounds, including ability to be erased (compromising authenticity of the records), smudging over time (resulting in illegibility), and unreliability of duplication by standard photo-optical methods. Inks should be fast-drying, solvent- and light-resistant, and "permanent" (stable over long-term storage and unreactive with paper). Aqueous-based inks are unacceptable because of potential smearing or obliteration upon contact with even small amounts of water. This is an important consideration—many popular contemporary pens (fountain pens, porous tip pens, and roller tip pens) commonly use water-based inks. Kanare has tested various inks and pen types and has studied relevant published performance standards (3). He concludes the following. A ball pen with black ink is best for all permanent scientific notekeeping. The decomposition (promoted by light) of colored inks is significant when compared with black ink. However, the usefulness of varying the color of inks such as when drawing diagrams may be essential in some types of work. Inventories of pens for laboratory use should only be sufficient for short-term (a few months) use. Long-term storage of ball-point pens is not advised because the ink component partitions within the ink cartridge and can result in problems of ink flow.

Notebook type

In academic institutions, there is a growing acceptance of the use of bound (sewn or glued binding) notebooks with serially numbered pages for recording data. In most (if not all) industrial research laboratories, however, such bound databooks are the standard. Kanare unequivocally states, "Plastic-bound books, wire-spiral books, and loose-leaf binders are not acceptable for writing permanent laboratory notes because pages can be intentionally inserted, removed, or accidentally ripped out." However, for reasons such as availability, convenience, and probably cost, loose-leaf notebooks historically have enjoyed popularity in research laboratories outside of the industrial setting.

Bound page-numbered databooks provide important features which comprise a compelling argument for their use. Their integral construction is consistent with preservation of data authenticity since intentional page deletion or insertion becomes immediately obvious. Quality control of paper composition in bound books is likely to be more consistent when compared with the vast array of papers available for loose-leaf books. Databooks of uniform size and shape also are more amenable to efficient and organized storage. Numbered volumes with serially numbered pages are easily indexed, making their task of locating stored data relatively easy. In sum, the keeping of bound databooks facilitates organization and ease of use that makes sense for the responsible custody of scientific data. Emphasis on scientific integrity and responsible scientific conduct has resulted in a heightened awareness of the importance of using bound notebooks in research laboratories. Additionally, the growing commercial applications of biomedical discoveries has further highlighted the importance of such laboratory tools. Finally, the pursuit of intellectual property protection—whether applying for or defending a patent—demands impeccable record keeping, which begins with the use of the proper databook.

Laboratory Record Keeping Policies

Principal investigators and laboratory leaders are well advised to develop standard policies for record keeping in their laboratories. The lack of policies or guidelines is a deficiency that is accentuated when new and inexperienced trainees or staff join the laboratory. Lack of such guidelines leads to problems with yet others in the lab who may be keeping records improperly. No guidance amounts to a tacit approval of slipshod practices that threaten the authenticity and integrity of scientific data. Ideas for developing such data keeping policies and practices can be obtained from a variety of sources including books (2,3) and some published lab manuals (1) and by contacting various industrial research laboratories or research institutes. The latter almost always have printed documents that cover record keeping and databook maintenance. Academic institutions usually don't have such guidelines or policies; indeed, the difficulties in covering widely divergent research areas makes the development of uniform policies impractical, if not impossible. On the other hand, programs or institutes within research universities can develop useful guidelines. For example, the Brain Tumor Research Center at the University of California, San Francisco has issued guidelines pertaining to research data collection and its management. Similarly, the Dana Farber Cancer Institute has policies for recording and preserving scientific data. Both of these documents may be found in the National Academy of Sciences volume *Responsible Science* (6).

Policy documents need not be complex or lengthy. They may reflect the experiences, training, and personal preferences of the principal investigator or group of principal investigators who write them. Group efforts are useful in writing guidelines, as the experience and wisdom of several investigators can provide a valuable perspective. Once in place, such documents should be regularly reviewed and modified as necessary. A clear statement about data ownership and retention should be part of such documents.

Suggestions for Record Keeping

Drawing from the references of the types cited in the previous section and from personal experience, the following provides an overview of laboratory record keeping practices useful in thinking about and developing specific policies.

Databooks

The case for using permanently bound laboratory notebooks with consecutively numbered pages has been made previously, but the discretion of the principal investigator should prevail ultimately in selecting specific notebook types and mandating their use. Hereafter in these discussions, use of bound databooks will be assumed. Some investigators like to control the distribution of databooks. For example, notebooks are given out as needed by the principal investigator or the lab manager. At the time of distribution, a record is made of the date, notebook user, and project; at this point the databook can be coded with a designation (e.g., a volume number or an alphanumeric identifier) which will allow for its tracking while in use or storage. This strategy has merit in laboratories where there are multiple trainees and staff working on a variety of projects, funded from different sources. Databook users should be clear on the lab policy for databook storage, retention in the lab, and any requirements for duplicating databook pages and other forms of data.

Organization

The first several pages of an individual's databook should be reserved for a table of contents. The first entry before beginning the table of contents should contain such basic information as the name of the databook user and, for work with potential proprietary implications, the location (room, building, institution) of the laboratory in which the experiments are being performed. Financial sponsorship should be identified by stating the title of the grant proposal, its agency identification number, dates of support, and the name of the principal investigator. Experiments listed in the table of contents should have concise but descriptive titles. Numbering experiments chronologically facilitates later cross-referencing. A glossary of abbreviations, symbols, or common designations may be included after the table of contents or, alternatively, can be listed at the end of the databook. Leave enough space for this information in order to be able to make additions to the glossary throughout the project.

The maintenance of a master databook log may be desirable. Such a central record (essentially a standard databook or perhaps even a computer-based word-processing or database algorithm) contains a listing of all experiments performed by the research team. Individuals are responsible for maintaining the log by entering experiment titles, dates, investigator names, and location of relevant data. A second type of laboratory-based reference resource is the methodology book. These books comprise a compendium of all standard laboratory methodology. Compilation of such books works best when it involves all laboratory members. Experimental methods should be described in sufficient detail to be useful even to the novice investigator. Electronic word processing makes this job easy. A printed copy of the complete book (in this case, loose-leaf or comparable binders are acceptable) can be kept in a central location, or duplicated copies (either printed or in electronic format) can be distributed to lab members. If a laboratory methods notebook is to be kept, it is critically important that the master copy, controlled by the principal investigator, be updated regularly—perhaps on an annual basis. Again, this can be a group effort, and will benefit by improvements and refinements of the individuals using the techniques. Updated copies of new methodology notebooks should be distributed to replace old versions. The previous version of the master methodology log, however, should be stored in an unaltered state. This is easily accomplished by creating an electronic (word processing) file. This allows for methods that have been updated or discontinued to be saved; referring back to methods, even discontinued ones, is sometimes necessary for a variety of reasons. Archiving such methods should be accomplished so that the date of revision or replacement of the method is obvious. Even where a central methodology book is maintained in the laboratory, it is a good idea for the databooks of individual investigators to contain descriptions of regularly used procedures. These can be transcribed directly, or typed copies can be prepared on high-quality paper which is then attached to the pages of the databook by using archival-quality tape or glue. Obviously, any specialized techniques or methods used in research projects (which might not be appropriate for a central methodology book) should be recorded in the individual's databook.

In a laboratory where strikingly different methods are used in various projects, a methods book may be kept separately by each member of the laboratory. In this case, investigators compile their own methods books and modify them as needed, leaving the original copy with the rest of their databooks when they leave the lab. All of the previously discussed considerations would apply to their maintenance. Modern biomedical research frequently involves methodologies and interdisciplinary research that requires the centralized organization of methods commonly used by the group. Such organization and maintenance facilitates the teaching of novice trainees and staff, assures quality control, and helps in the troubleshooting of technical problems. However, decisions relating to whether to use a centralized or decentralized method of record keeping should be made by the laboratory leader.

Tangible data and the databook
Items such as photographs, negatives, autoradiograms, printouts, and other tangible forms of data should be included in the databook where this is physically possible. The use of archival-quality glues and tapes is suggested for affixing such materials to databooks. Materials that cannot be glued or taped directly into the book should be inserted into plastic sleeves which are then fixed in the databook. Printed material, especially that produced by photocopying or laser printing, should not come in contact with plastic material of any type. Over time the ink will transfer its image to the plastic and this will obscure, if not ruin, the printed data. Information which is collected on tape, printouts, thermofax paper, or any paper stock of low quality should be photocopied onto high-quality paper before gluing or taping into the databook.

Certain materials that contain or represent data cannot be practically included in the laboratory databook. These include, for example, oversize photographic or autoradiographic material, magnetic media, embedded specimens or tissues, or some data obtained by light or electron microscopy. Proper storage of such materials should take into account such factors as humidity, temperature, light, security, and ease of accessibility. For example, oversize X-ray films contained in protective sleeves which are appropriately coded can be stored in metal cabinets of some type. Pressed board boxes also are useful for storage. Such containers come in varied sizes and shapes, but only those composed of acid-free materials should be used. Ordinary cardboard boxes, even those commercially sold for storage purposes, are inferior and can release damaging acids over time. When remote site storage is used, it is important that a description of the data storage system, the storage location, and the coding scheme be described in one's laboratory notebook. As a rule, an individual who inspects the databook should be able to locate all forms of data relevant to the experiments presented simply by reading its pages. If centrally stored data (e.g., electron microsope grids or autoradiograms) cannot be located by reading the databook, then repeating certain experiments or observations may not be possible.

For maximum longevity, prolonged storage of databooks and related materials such as photographs, negatives, or oversized documents should ideally occur under conditions of controlled temperature (68 ± 3°F) and relative humidity (<50%). Basements, attics, and poorly ventilated storage rooms are notoriously bad places for long-term storage of data and databooks.

Format

Investigators should create a standard plan that details the way in which experiments will be recorded in the databook. Honesty and accuracy are critical. Some argue that writing should be concise. Although this is a reasonable guiding principle, it should never compromise the capturing of any part of an experiment. For example, if an observation requires an explanation which is complex and must be described at extraordinary length, then this should be done without reservation. The same is true for interpretations and for thoughts on plans for additional work. The databook is arguably the place where the investigator's physical and mental activities related to experimentation are recorded. Presentation and detail must be complete, comprehensible, and legible.

Purpose. Each description should begin with a brief but instructive statement of the purpose of the experiment. This is done no matter how routine the experiment. Whether the experiment is to test some elegant hypothesis or simply to isolate cellular DNA, a purpose should be articulated. No experiment is too trivial to not warrant a written purpose. For example, at some point an investigator might want to know how many independently isolated preparations of a plasmid were used in performing genetic mapping studies. His or her job is simplified if each preparative run can be traced to a clearly recorded experiment that begins with a statement of purpose. As a key element of format, the statement of purpose facilitates navigating through databooks.

Materials and methods. A description of any methodology not found in the laboratory central methods manual should be included in the databook. The appropriate literature from which methods are derived should be cited. Assuming a central methods book exists as described previously, methods used may be cited by referring back to the central laboratory source book. Specific reference to the exact book (likely designated by date, e.g., "1994 version") should be made so that the precise method may be located in the future. If there are deviations from the referenced procedure, such changes must be precisely indicated. To eliminate any confusion, it may be necessary to write the modified method in the databook.

The materials and methods section of the experiment should also document materials being used. The grade, sources, and lot numbers of specialized chemicals, reagents, and enzymes should all be recorded. If there is any question about the name recognition of the supplier (e.g., supplier of a rare chemical or unusual enzyme), the name, address, and phone number of that supplier should be included. In the case of biological materials such as cell lines, bacterial strains, or animals, specific information on properties (e.g., genotypes and phenotypes) and source should be recorded. If working laboratory designations have been used for convenience, a full explanation of the original designation should be included.

Each repeat of an experiment should be written up separately in the databook. For materials and methods, it is acceptable to record the information with appropriate detail and completeness the first time the experiment is performed. Assuming no changes in methodology are implemented in future runs, it is acceptable to refer back to the materials and methods section recorded in the first experiment of the series. If changes are made, reference to the original methods can be made and the modifications noted. When recording changes made to established or previously tried protocols, it is a good idea to present the rationale for the change. Necessary modifications tried at one point in time might not be obvious to databook users several months later.

If an experiment requires the use of specialized equipment, relevant information should be recorded in the databook. For example, if several electron microscopes are available for the work, which one (type, location) was used in the experiment? If calibration of a piece of hardware is required, information on the calibration process should be recorded as well.

Observations and results. Data should be entered directly into the databook as soon as they become available. Original data recorded in handscript are always entered directly into the databook. Data should never be written on loose sheets of paper and then transcribed later into the databook. This practice risks the incorporation of errors durng transcription and may compromise the authenticity of the data. Direct recording of data requires organization at two levels. First, any writing that will facilitate data entry should be planned and carried out in advance of doing the experiment. For example, a matrix drawn and labeled to receive written data from instrument readings greatly assists data collection. The second organizational consideration involves the physical availability of the databook to the investigator while the experiment is being performed. The databook should always be conveniently accessible to the investigator. This may mean arranging bench work space ahead of time to accommodate the physical tools of the experiment, including the databook itself.

In addition to recorded data, the observations and results section should contain all renderings of the data, including calculations (with explanation) and organized presentations such as resulting tables and graphs. Tables and graphs should be clearly labeled. Photographic materials should be affixed to the page by using archival glue or tape. Any related materials not included in the databook should be catalogued and their storage location identified. For example, photographs attached to the databook may have their corresponding negatives stored in an appropriate file (see below). Negatives should be contained in glassine envelopes and stored at room temperature away from sources of high humidity, excessive light, and temperature variability (i.e., avoid proximity to windows, water baths, incubators, ovens, or autoclaves).

Discussion. Each experiment should be discussed following the recording of observations and calculations. It may be necessary to enter discussion comments at various places in the experimental write-up. In other words, the discussion for a single experiment need not be organized to appear at the conclusion of the write-up. It is appropriate to include comments that capture impressions and present interpretations at various places in the written experiment. This is convenient and ensures the most effective use of space in the databook itself. The standard format presentation usually required by scientific journals, with its clear separation of the actual results and their discussion, is not usually applied to databook keeping.

The last entry in the completed write-up of the experiment should state the conclusions of the work. This should be done, even if it is repeats previously written comments. Conclusions logically belong at the end of the experiment. Just as we look to the beginning of the write-up of an experiment to find a purpose, conclusions are logically sought at the end of the write-up. A conclusion should be written no matter how trivial or routine it is thought to be. Future reference to the databook is aided by written experiments that have a clear beginning and a clear end.

There is no clear agreement about acceptable style of the discussion section. Much debate has centered around the appropriateness of comments that editorialize on results. Some investigators urge refraining from this on the grounds that it may create confusion and mislead others at a later time. Moreover, it is generally inconsistent with the overall recommendation of recording notes in as concise a fashion as possible. Others argue that the databook should record all of the mental and physical activities of the investigator. Accordingly, if something is important enough to record, then a note of it should be made. Interestingly, some industrial research databook policies admonish investigators to never make comments that could be subject to misinterpretation by others. Specifically, investigators are cautioned against using phraseology like "the experiment failed" or describing a yield of some biological material as "no good." This is argued on the theoretical grounds that far-reaching conclusions ought not be based on the interpretation of a single experiment. Repetition and confirmation are always necessary and hence subjective statements about individual experiments are considered ill advised and are vulnerable to incorrect interpretation. In practice, such statements are potentially damaging to a planned or existing intellectual property position (e.g., a patent application).

Good databook keeping

For single projects (e.g., a dissertation research project), databooks should be used consecutively; multiple databooks are best avoided. Once appropriate pages are reserved for a table of contents and abbreviation list (if necessary), data should be recorded in a continuous and chronological fashion with no intervening pages. Each experiment and the entry of all recorded data and comments should be dated individually. Many suggest writing each page in such a way that little or no margin space is available for after-the-fact note taking. If an alternative explanation of the data becomes apparent, one should begin a new entry at the next available point in the databook and cross-reference the new entry with the original experiment (page and experiment number). Unused portions of any databook pages should be marked through with pen. This helps in the visual organization of a databook that may include specific experiments interspersed with general note taking related to other experiments.

Mistakes in the databook should be marked through with a single line and a full explanation of the error provided. For mistakes made that can be corrected instantly, this practice presents no problem with available page space. For mistakes discovered at a later date, there may not be enough space to provide an explanation. Thus, an investigator would mark a line through the error and write: "See page XX for explanation." Never obliterate mistakes with ink or cover them with any type of correcting fluid. Their legibility may be important later, as such incorrect entries may provide needed information. Additionally, to the casual observer, practices that appear to remove data from the databook may suggest improper motivation.

Witnessing of data and interactions with other people. Witnessing of data is a required procedure in the industrial research laboratory. The need to protect inventions and potentially patentable ideas necessitates this practice. Witnessing of data is far less common, however, in the academic research laboratory. An exception might be a requirement by a funding agency for certain types of contract work (e.g., clinical testing). However, little thought is generally given to witnessing the databooks produced during the course of most basic research projects comprising thesis or dissertation research. Investigators performing fundamental experiments don't often think about their work leading directly or indirectly to a discovery of a commercial application that would require the protection of a patent. However, the unexpected bridging of basic and applied research is becoming commonplace in the biomedical sciences. Witnessing of data is necessary if the work may lead to a patentable discovery or invention. In the academic or basic research institute where rules for witnessing don't usually exist, establishment and enforcement of such a policy resides with the laboratory director. In deciding to put such a policy in place, the investigator must consider the requirements (if any) of funding agencies and the potential for applied science emerging from the research.

Where it is a standard practice in research laboratories, each and every page of the databook is witnessed. The witness who signs and dates the page of the databook being examined must be able to understand the work. The signature may be accompanied by a declaration that says "witnessed and understood." Many commercially available databooks have this declaration and a line or box for signature and date printed on each page. The witness must not be a co-inventor. In patent prosecution, co-inventors are not allowed to corroborate each other's work. Thus, selection of a neutral party who is able to understand the work is needed for appropriate witnessing of scientific data. Consider, for example, a discovery that grew from a predoctoral research project. The trainee's mentor would likely be considered a co-inventor and, thus, should not sign as a witness to the data. Another worker in the same lab could sign, assuming they understood the work but were not involved in it.

A databook witness may be called on to testify in the prosecution or defense of a patent. Witnesses corroborate the timing of events and must be able to understand ideas and the experimental basis of their formation. They must have a clear understanding of the assignment of credit: Whose idea was it, anyway? Failure to observe the proper criteria for selecting databook witnesses can undermine or nullify claims on intellectual property.

It is desirable to record in the databook discussions with others about the research. Such notes should list the names of the individuals talked to, along with the time and relevant points of the discussion. This is a good record keeping habit that will help trace the investigator's thinking processes and provides a prompt when it is time to attribute credit. In addition, should corroboration of data be needed at some point, tracking down individuals who can talk about certain of the experiments is the next best thing to a witnessed databook page.

Correspondence to and from colleagues about experiments should be recorded in the databook as well. Letters can be photocopied on high-quality paper and then fixed in the notebook by using archival tape or glue. Alternatively, it may be appropriate to make notes from such correspondence in the notebook and then refer to the location of the letter in a file that can be easily found later by someone reading the notebook.

Finally, names and roles of individuals who have played any part in the research need be entered in the databook along with a description of their contributions. Collaborative researchers fall into this category. Agreements with collaborators pertaining to research contributions, expenditures of grants, personnel involvement, and perhaps most importantly, authorship on papers should be recorded in the databook. People who have participated in one's research even on a fee-for-service basis should be noted. Technicians working in institutional core laboratories are especially important. Who made the oligonucleotide or hybridoma or ran the automated DNA sequencer for the experiment? These notations represent a record of quality control. They can help in troubleshooting problems and can provide a source of independent corroboration in matters of intellectual property.

Electronic record keeping. The use of free-standing or networked personal computers will eventually play a major role in research laboratory record keeping. There are several advantages to such techniques. Clarity and organization are facilitated by keyboard input, and the entry of graphs, tables, and photographic material can be accomplished using software (drawing, graphing, and data analysis programs) as well as scanners that can digitize hand-drawn materials. Access to electronic data can be managed using passwords or controlled accounts and this provides a security advantage while at the same time allowing more efficient access to data by authorized individuals. (For example, mentors could check trainees' data stored in the memory of a central computer hard drive.) Enormous amounts of electronic data can be stored in a very small space compared with traditional lab databooks, and accessing experimental protocols and data by electronic searching is powerful and rapid.

Disadvantages to electronic record keeping exist as well. Witnessing an electronic databook "page" is open to question. Although scanning technology and automated handwriting digitizers can provide the means to do this, the legal acceptance of such methods has not yet been tested. Another disadvantage that will likely be overcome is the inclusion of an unalterable time and date record associated with the data. Techniques to do this have been developed and are being applied. Digital "time stamping" programs are being used as well, but these usually require that an independent party collect and maintain records. This logistical problem makes the utility of such programs impractical for the typical academic or basic research lab.

The use of the computer in laboratory record keeping is currently in transition. "Laboratory notebook" software programs are coming onto the market, but their usefulness, especially in research work of proprietary or commercial nature, has been largely untested in both practical and legal senses. In contrast, the use of computers to prepare charts, graphs, and other forms of data analysis is growing rapidly. Such data, however, should always be printed on suitable paper and affixed to the pages of a bound databook.

A final word. Notes prepared in advance of an oral presentation can take two general forms. The first includes short phrases, words, or occasional sentences that trigger a speaker's memory. The second form is a verbatim text of the speaker's remarks—a script of every word he or she will speak. There are no abbreviations, cryptic reminders, or shorthand notations. If the speaker were suddenly taken ill, a colleague could easily give the speech if it were prepared in the latter form. However, it is doubtful that a substitute could successfully deliver the speech with only the abbreviated notes. Similarly, a laboratory databook is inherently more useful as the "verbatim text" of experimental work. In his book *The Cuckoo's Egg* (Doubleday, New York, 1989), Clifford Stoll lauds the value of a carefully documented logbook. His advice rings true as an axiom of scientific record keeping: "If you don't document it, you might as well not have observed it."

Information on Supplies for Record Keeping

A principal supplier of bound notebooks suitable for laboratory record keeping is the Avery-Dennison Company of Framingham, Massachusetts [(508) 879-0511]. The company will supply information on the type of laboratory notebooks ("computation notebooks") they have, but they do not sell directly to individuals. Instead, they distribute their products through office supply companies, stationary retailers, and university bookstores. Their notebooks come in several standard formats. The paper contained in most of their products is of high quality but is not acid-free.

Some companies specialize in databook manufacturing. Products marketed by these companies contain acid-free paper and come in standard or custom-designed formats. These companies do sell directly to individual customers, but usually require minimum orders. Some of their databooks are carried by university bookstores.

For standard format databooks of varying styles:

Scientific Notebook Company

P.O. Box 238

Stevensville, MI 49127

Phone: (616) 429-8285

For custom-manufactured databooks:

Eureka Blank Book Company

P.O. Box 150

Holyoke, MA 01041-0150

Phone: (413) 534-5671

Laboratory Notebook Company

P.O. Box 188

Holyoke, MA 01041-0188

Phone: (413) 532-6287

Materials for archiving, including acid-free glue, archival mending tape, and acid-free boxes of varying styles and sizes are sold by:

University Products, Inc.

517 Main Street

P.O. Box 101

Holyoke, MA 01041-0101

Phone: (800) 762-1165

The West Coast distributor for University Products, Inc., is:

Conservation Materials, Ltd.

240 Freeport Blvd.

Sparks, NV 89431

Phone: (702) 331-0582

Case Studies

3.1 A predoctoral student working in the laboratory of her mentor is gathering data for a federally funded project on which the mentor serves as principal investigator. The student is, of course, going to use the data for her dissertation work. The student and mentor have a terrible falling out. The student leaves the lab and finds a new advisor. The advisor notices that data and materials related to the student's project are missing. The student readily admits to removing the tissue sections, gels, and computer disks but asserts that they are "hers"— the product of her sweat and blood. What issues of data ownership apply here and what should be done?

3.2 A graduate student, working on a project that involves extensive DNA sequencing, provides his mentor with a computer-generated sequence of a gene. The student tells his mentor that the sequence determination has involved complete analysis of both strands of the DNA molecule. Over the next several months, it is determined that not all of the sequence data reflect analysis of both DNA strands. Indeed, follow-up work by a postdoctoral in the laboratory reveals several mistakes in the sequence. The student in question admits to misleading his mentor and, following appropriate investigation, is convicted of scientific misconduct and dismissed from the graduate program. The mentor realizes that the student presented some of the erroneous data at a regional scientific meeting. Proceedings of the meeting were not published, but abstracts of all of the works presented were distributed to approximately 100 meeting participants. In addition, the student (with the mentor's permission) sent the sequence by electronic mail to three other laboratories. What, if any, responsibility does the faculty mentor have with regard to disclosing the above developments? What, if anything, should the mentor do about the prematurely released data? Under these circumstances, what is the potential for harm coming from this incident of scientific fraud? Who might be harmed?

3.3 The research laboratory of a faculty investigator has begun using a new electrophoresis technique. The technique works well in the hands of the laboratory investigators. A field service representative from the company that manufactures the apparatus asks several of the workers in the laboratory if he may borrow some of the photographs of their results to show to potential clients. In return, he offers to take the whole lab to dinner at an expensive restaurant. The lab members comply and the whole group goes to dinner a few weeks later. You, as laboratory director, are told of this entire series of events after the fact. Comment on the data ownership and laboratory record keeping implications of this scenario. What action, if any, is necessary on the mentor's part?

3.4 You are present during a conversation in the departmental conference room. Jim, a new assistant professor, is getting ready to submit his first paper since joining the faculty. He reviews one of the figures, which is a photo of an ethidium bromide-stained agarose gel. The gel contains the products of polymerase chain reaction-amplified whole cell DNA. The photo displays the predicted 3-kb DNA fragment. Jim comments that a second minor signal was also evident on the original gel. Based on its size, Jim believes that this second fragment represents a very exciting discovery, but it needs considerable additional work. This second fragment cannot be seen in the photograph. Jim discloses that this is because he has deliberately prepared an overexposed print in order to obscure the second fragment. He says he did this because he is worried that competing groups in larger, more established labs will interpret the potential of the second fragment and will "scoop" him. He has prepared a figure legend that says "a second minor signal of unexplained origin was present in this experiment but is not visible in the photo," but the figure legend does not include the size of the unexplained fragment. Thus, he argues he'll be telling the truth while at the same time protecting himself from his competition. Are Jim's actions appropriate? Is he (1) simply playing fairly in the hotly competitive arena of biomedical research, or (2) falling victim to self-deception, or (3) perpetrating scientific fraud?

3.5 You have submitted a manuscript to a peer-reviewed journal. It contains primary nucleotide sequence data for a new gene as well as its upstream sequences. When you receive the paper back from the editor, it is accompanied by two favorable reviews written by expert *ad hoc* referees. One of the referees has some suggestions regarding the interpretation of your sequence data. Specifically the reviewer attaches a new printout of your entire sequence data with some computer-generated structures. These represent predictions of folded messenger RNA derived from the transcription of your gene. The reviewer's interpretations have implications for translational genetic control of the gene. It is clear to you that the reviewer has made an electronic file of your sequence data and has subjected the data to his or her own analysis. Did the reviewer do anything wrong in your view? Will you discuss this with the editor of the journal? If so, what inquiries, comments, or requests will you direct to the editor?

3.6 Bob, your fellow predoctoral graduate student, comes to you for advice. Bob's mentor recently has noticed that he keeps his stained, desiccated polyacrylamide gels in sealed plastic bags that are taped to the pages of his databook. Bob considers such gels to be primary data that must be retained in their original form. Bob's mentor has ordered him to stop doing this. Moreover, he tells Bob to remove the gels already in his databook. Bob's mentor says that polyacrylamide is a neurotoxin and should be disposed of properly. Further, he tells Bob to make black and white photographs of all his previous gels and to retain both the print and negative for each gel. He says that in the future, this practice should be followed for all acrylamide gel data storage. He says the photos are to be considered the primary data and retained in Bob's databook. Bob disagrees with his mentor and argues that photographs can be altered and that a desiccated gel is an accurate representation of the original data. He also argues that once the acrylamide is sealed in plastic, there is no danger of exposure to toxic material. Bob's mentor dismisses these arguments and gives him one month to photograph the existing gels and to dispose of them. Bob is very upset. He thinks his mentor is acting irresponsibly with respect to data retention. He also feels his mentor is being a bully in forcing him to adopt his own personal preferences. What advice do you give Bob? Should Bob seek additional advice from another faculty member or the departmental chair?

3.7 You meet a colleague at a national meeting who is working in your field. You exchange information on your research and he agrees to send you a diskette containing the amino acid sequence of a protein, called *XYZ*. The nucleotide sequence of the gene encoding this protein was determined in his lab but has not been published. You return from the meeting and the diskette is in your mail as promised. You are fascinated by the sequence and suggest that one of your students analyze it. The student proceeds to analyze XYZ by using computer algorithms and prepares several printouts of amino acid sequence comparisons with proteins being studied in your lab. The student's results are exciting and you ask her to make a presentation at a journal club involving your research group and those of three other faculty members. The student does so. Following the meeting, a faculty colleague in attendance at the presentation accompanies you back to your office and asks to speak with you privately. He questions how you obtained the data and indicates concern that your student has disclosed privileged information without permission. He claims this is particularly problematic because the data have not appeared in print and you did not seek specific permission to have the data discussed in an open forum. Further, he expresses concern that your new findings on the amino acid sequence of XYZ should have been shared immediately with the investigator who provided you with the data. How do you respond to your faculty colleague?

3.8 A predoctoral trainee under your supervision has had several difficult years finishing up his dissertation research. He has needed continual guidance, and his attitude has not been positive about the work. He does not seem motivated, but you press him almost on a daily basis until the work is completed and the dissertation is finally written. The student turns in an average defense and informs you that he is leaving science to take a job in biomedical sales. Several areas of the student's dissertation need additional work before the research can be written up for publication. You turn several portions of the dissertation work over to a competent postdoctoral trainee in your laboratory. Over the course of the next several weeks, the postdoctoral pursues these new lines of experimentation. In the process, however, she uncovers several problems with the data in the dissertation. In fact, a number of experiments cannot be repeated. Moreover, some of the results obtained are opposite those reported in the student's dissertation. These results have serious implications regarding interpretations and conclusions reached by the student in his dissertation. You review the student's databooks and are unable to find entries that could have been used to construct some of the tables seen in the dissertation. Moreover, other data sets written into the databook have been used selectively to construct some tables in the dissertation (i.e., critical points that would have confused analysis were omitted). After considerable analysis and discussion with the postdoctoral, you decide that the student has at least falsified data and possibly fabricated data presented in his dissertation. You have not yet published any of the work of the student's dissertation in manuscript form. However, one published abstract contains accurate information which has been authenticated by your postdoctoral trainee. All of the student's work was supported by your NIH grant. What actions(s), if any, do you take in this situation?

REFERENCES

1. **Becker, J., G. A. Caldwell, and E. A. Zachgo.** *Biotechnology—A Laboratory Course.* Academic Press, San Diego, CA.
2. **Grisson, F., and D. Pressman.** 1987. *The Inventor's Notebook.* Nolo Press, Berkeley, CA.
3. **Kanare, H. M.** 1985. *Writing the Laboratory Notebook.* American Chemical Society, Washington, D.C.
4. **Rayl, A. J. S.** 1991. Misconduct case stresses importance of good notekeeping. *Scientist,* November 11, p. 18–20.
5. **U.S. Department of Health and Human Services, Public Health Service.** 1990. PHS Grants Policy Statement Sec. 2–3. DHHS Publication No. (OASH) 90-50,000 (Rev.), October 1.
6. **U.S. National Academy of Sciences.** 1993. *Responsible Science,* Vol. II: *Ensuring the Integrity of the Research Process,* p. 203–205, 206–222. National Academy Press, Washington, D.C.

4 | *Authorship and Peer Review*

Francis L. Macrina

Scientific Publication and Authorship

Publication of experimental work accomplishes several things. It allows evaluation of results and places them in perspective against a larger body of knowledge. It also credits other scientists, whose contributions and ideas have been used and built upon in the research. It enables others to extend or repeat work by providing a description of experiments performed. Finally, the author byline attributes credit for the work and, perhaps most importantly, establishes who accepts responsibility for it.

Scientists, their professional societies, and the publishers and editors of scholarly journals all agree that the determination of authorship is an important matter. In general, authors must contribute to the reported work in some way; what ultimately gets recognized as an appropriate contribution varies, however. Defining the responsibilities of authorship thus represents an even larger problem. Suppose a published paper contains an honest mistake that has a major effect on the paper's scientific message. It is determined that the mistake is attributable to one of the four coauthors on the paper. Are the other three authors responsible for the mistake as well? Or, does their responsibility simply stop with an adequate explanation of why they couldn't have detected it? If it is determined that the "mistake" was the result of some fraudulent behavior on the part of just one coauthor, are the answers to these questions still the same?

Historically, the scientific community has relied on rather informal, often unwritten, and sometimes ill-defined criteria for determining authorship on scientific papers. This approach has not served science well. It can breed misunderstanding, hard feelings, and confusion among the scientists affected by such decisions. The current climate, however, is changing as institutions, societies, editorial boards, and publishers seek to clarify and even codify the criteria used to assign authorship and its related responsibilities. Interestingly, this has occurred in spite of occasional arguments that attempts to formally address this issue impose on academic freedom and stifle creativity.

The Need for Authorship Criteria

Scientists concur that it would be wrong to include as an author on a paper someone who had made no experimental, technical, or intellectual contributions to the work. Similarly, if an investigator performed a key experiment and provided an interpretation of the results, authorship for that person would be obligatory. These extremes have never really been in question, and they can be correctly decided without hesitation. But, unfortunately, the day-to-day decisions on authoring scientific papers fall in between these examples. And the questions of the responsibility of individuals whose names appear on multi-authored papers remain largely unanswered, although they are increasingly debated. "If you are willing to take the credit, you have to take the responsibility" is a much used statement that is not as straightforward as one would think in every case of coauthored scientific publications. Many now insist that guidelines, if not policies, are needed which deal with deciding on authorship and defining responsibilities.

The Pressure To Publish

Humanistic realities are superimposed on the practices and standards of scientific publication. Regardless of the setting in which scientific research occurs, publications have become a stock in trade. In academic settings, publications help scientists win grants, promotions, tenure, higher salaries, and professional prestige. For these reasons, there is pressure to publish. Unfortunately, some scientists react to these pressures in ways that lead to irresponsible actions. Temptations to do this abound, and succumbing to them can be easy to rationalize. The need for that "one additional paper" for the progress report of a grant application (to get a grant award), or an employer's activity report (to get a raise), or one's curriculum vitae (to get a job) creates pressure to publish. Even if the data are incomplete, there always seems to be some opportunity to publish. The large and growing number of journals in scientific disciplines provides many options for submitting papers. Journal quality and reviewing standards vary so there is likely to be someplace the research can be published.

The temptation to publish incomplete work also crops up as a result of another type of pressure: the need to be "first." To keep research funding scientists must be productive, and prestige in science is often associated with being on "the cutting edge" of the field. Publishing quickly advertises research progress and the pressures to do this sometimes lead to compromises. Finally, there are a number of other reasons that lead to questionable publication practices. Rationalizations abound, such as, "We didn't know what to make of the data so we got them out into the literature so others might evaluate them"; or, "It was the last set of results from her dissertation research and didn't seem to fit in the other manuscripts so we published it independently."

These pressures to publish have given rise to euphemisms that describe what sometimes happens in scientific publishing. "Salami science" refers to the publication of related results in "slices": data sets are split and published separately instead of being presented in a unified way. This increases the number of published papers from the same amount of data, giving the impression of increased productivity. Another phrase used to describe a related practice is "the least publishable unit," or the smallest amount of data that can be written as a manuscript and published. Some publications and editors may be unconsciously contributing to these practices. Publication categories termed "Notes," "Short Communications," or "Preliminary Reports" usually accept brief reports of important findings that can stand on their own (the language varies, but the message is the same). When editors and reviewers do not heed their journal's policies, such brief publication formats open the door to the "salami slicers" and the "reductionists." The ethics of publishing results in a way to maximize the number of papers is open to debate. Most would argue that it is not inherently wrong and scientists must have the freedom to publish how and what they see fit. However, the fragmentary nature of these publications sometimes makes them difficult to evaluate. They can mislead the reader and create confusion in the field by giving inappropriate emphasis to a piece of work. Additionally, unjustified multiple publications put undue strain on the peer review process.

Authorship and its responsibilities need to be better defined. In biomedical research, interdisciplinary approaches to problems breed collaboration. This makes multiauthorship the norm, and there is no expectation that the number of coauthors has to be limited. Thus, single-authored research papers have become a rarity. Even at the most fundamental of all levels—the training of students and postdoctorals—the multiauthored paper is appropriate and expected. Mentors and trainees both have a stake in their published work. Defining that stake can be elusive, however, without rational guidelines. Sorting out details, identifying acceptable criteria, and monitoring policies has not been easy. But developing usable guidelines, no matter how "flexible" or "open-ended," is the responsibility of the scientific community.

This chapter reviews some of the commonly accepted standards of publication and authorship, including the process and responsibilities associated with the peer review of a scientific publication.

Instructions to Authors

Some of the standards for authorship and publication are readily accessible to the novice author. These appear on what may be the least read pages of a scientific journal: the "Instructions to Authors" section. The instructions to authors published in scientific journals provide the details of manuscript preparation required by the journal, its general policies, and often its philosophy of publication (i.e., standards for publication). Sometimes these issues are reaffirmed after the paper is submitted; for example, they may be stated in the letter acknowledging receipt of the manuscript, the acceptance letter, or in material sent with page proofs. Instructions to authors should always be read before beginning manuscript preparation. In fact, consulting these instructions provide guidance when deciding upon which journal to publish in. Journal publishers often use this space to state the kinds of research considered appropriate for publication. This information, along with experience and observation of the published material that appears in the journal, helps with the decision on where to submit a paper. In addition, it is helpful to seek the advice of experienced colleagues on where the work might be best published. Instructions to authors appear in every issue of some journals. In others, they appear periodically, but reference to their location is published somewhere in every issue.

Details of manuscript preparation

Instructions to authors contain essential information needed to prepare and submit the manuscript. Details on format, space constraints or word limitations, figure preparation, the use of abbreviations and symbols, and proper chemical, biological, and genetic nomenclature are found therein. For symbol and nomenclature information, many journals use varying authoritative reference books or guides as their accepted standards. Instructions to authors often contain housekeeping details such as how many copies to submit, where to mail the manuscript, and, where appropriate, the cost of page charges. Finally, some journals provide guidance on the preparation of the various sections of the scientific paper: the abstract, introduction, materials and methods, results, and discussion. Such guidance is useful to the novice writer. Reading the journal's guidelines on how to prepare these sections is preferable to trying to deduce them from reading papers published in the journal (although this can help too).

Authorship

Some journals more or less define authorship and its responsibilities. The words ultimately boil down to the same two issues in the vast majority of examples. First, an author has to make a significant contribution to the work. Most statements like this leave plenty of room for interpretation, and thus are flexible (a trait favored by some and opposed by others). Second, statements defining authorship often mention that all authors on a manuscript take responsibility for its content. With multiauthored papers, statements are occasionally included that indicate that all of the authors consent to its submission, or that they all have read the manuscript. Such statements have important meaning in setting the stage for the broader issues of authorship responsibility.

Copyright

A usual condition of manuscript acceptance for almost all, if not all, scientific journals is that the authors assign the copyright to the publisher (this is discussed in more detail in Chapter 8). Usually the senior author (sometimes called the corresponding author) is empowered to do this for all coauthors. Also, many journals require that authors obtain permission to use any copyrighted material that is included in their manuscript (for example, a diagram from a previously published paper). This is usually a formality that involves writing the publisher who holds the copyright for the work to be included. The letter should describe the intended use of the copyrighted material. Many publishers have forms that can be completed in lieu of a letter.

Manuscript review

Matters relating to the peer review of the manuscript often are found in the Instructions to Authors text. Some journals allow authors to suggest the names of impartial reviewers, either *ad hoc* referees or members of the editorial board. This assists the editors with their job and it is wise to take advantage of the opportunity where it exists. In this context, who qualifies as an impartial reviewer? Opinions vary and criteria are subjective. Often excluded as impartial reviewers are (1) people at the author's institution, (2) people who have been associated with the author's laboratory, and (3) the author's collaborators or coauthors at other institutions. Individuals in the latter two categories are considered in view of the time period that has elapsed since the author's last interactions with them. Such things must be evaluated on a case-by-case basis. Potential conflict of interest related to the suggestion of peer reviewers is often best determined by the author. Common indicators of conflict of interest are manifest in one's spending inordinate amounts of time rationalizing suggestions for a reviewer, or an uneasiness that comes with discussing proposed reviewers with other colleagues.

Often a description of the peer view process is found in the Instructions to Authors section. The process also may be described in the letter or card that acknowledges receipt of the manuscript. Authors need to become familiar with this process and understand how it works. It can vary significantly for different journals. Understanding the process will facilitate handling of the manuscript during peer review. The typical path of a manuscript through the review process will be presented later in this chapter.

Prior publication

The varied Instructions to Authors sections are usually quite explicit about the issue of prior publication. Work may not be submitted that has been previously published or has been submitted to another journal. One publisher has invoked the concept of the primary scientific publication to help clarify this issue. Robert Day in his book *How to Write and Publish a Scientific Paper* (4th edition) defines the primary publication as ..."(*i*) the first publication of original research results, (*ii*) in a form whereby peers of the author can repeat the experiments and test the conclusions, and (*iii*) in a journal or other source document readily available within the scientific community."

However, most would argue that issues of prior publication are far from straightforward. Ambiguity frequently exists when considering, for example, papers published in monographs (e.g., invited short papers or meeting proceedings). It is not easy to determine how "readily available" a source may be. How many copies of a monograph have to be sold or distributed in order for it to fall into this category? If all copies of the monograph have been distributed in the United States, is it acceptable to submit essentially the same work to a journal published in Europe? Some argue that original work published in conference reports, symposia or meeting proceedings, or the equivalent monographs is by definition preliminary due to considerations of format and space. Often methods cannot be fully described. They also argue that such work is usually not subjected to peer review. The potential for self-deception is large, however, and scientists generally agree it is wrong to publish the same material as a primary publication in two different places. Using that philosophy as a guide is highly recommended.

Unpublished information cited in manuscripts
Some journals require proof of permission to cite the unpublished work of others. Thus, information provided by a colleague as a "personal communication" may require a letter granting permission. The same may be true for preprints or submitted manuscripts provided by one's colleagues. This practice is increasing among publishers of scientific journals. Such language mandates formal communication among scientists and can avoid potential problems. For example, a colleague might provide a manuscript that has been submitted for publication, but she may not feel comfortable allowing the work to be cited in another paper before she knows whether it has been accepted. By formally asking her permission, any prospect of misunderstanding is eliminated.

Regarding the author's unpublished work—"in press" or "submitted" manuscripts—an increasing number of journals require that copies of such manuscripts accompany the new submission so that they can be used if needed during peer review.

Sharing research materials

In natural science and biomedical journals, it has become standard for publishers to include statements about sharing research materials. This includes cell lines, microorganisms, mutants, plasmids, antibodies, and other biologicals or reagents. There are usually conditions stated for the release of such materials. For example, materials must be available at cost (e.g., preparation and shipping), they must be requested in reasonable quantities, and they must not be used for commercial purposes. Scientists also usually observe the practice of requesting materials from the authors of the publication in which the material was initially described. For example, it is not acceptable to request a bacterial strain from a third party, even though it may be convenient to do that. A mutant critically needed for work in Chicago may have been constructed by a scientist in Japan, but may already be in the possession of a colleague in a nearby city. It is not appropriate to ask the stateside colleague to provide the mutant. One should ask the Japanese investigator who originally constructed it and published the results. At the very least, you might suggest that he allow you to get a culture from your conveniently located neighbor.

The sharing of research materials might also be mandated by author's instructions that request that authors properly deposit specialized data in appropriate databases (e.g., nucleic acid sequences and X-ray crystallographic data). The exchange of research materials and the proper deposition of results into databases are usually listed as conditions of acceptance for the paper.

Conflict of interest

Scientific journals may ask authors to disclose their financial associations with companies whose activities might be affected by the results of the paper. If the paper is accepted, this disclosure is usually handled on a case-by-case basis. Potential conflict of interest disclosure is, however, likely to become a more prominent issue as research sponsored by the biotechnology industry continues to increase in academic institutions and in noncommercial research institutes. Thus far, related language in author's instructions has been found primarily in biomedical journals that publish research with clinical implications. Other related issues will undoubtedly have to addressed. For example, what about parallel conflicts involving members of editorial boards who serve as reviewers for such papers? What about editors themselves who may have financial associations with companies whose activities may overlap with the content of journal articles? Is that conflict of interest, real or perceived? How can such issues be monitored and how are conflicts handled when they are identified? There are no ready answers, but the need for dialogue, careful consideration, and the development and implementation of policies is apparent.

Imperfections

Some journals also include policies on the handling of disputes once papers are published. Occasionally, journals are explicit about the option of having their editors examine original data in the process of dispute resolution. In addition, many journals describe policies for publishing corrections, errata, or retractions of papers.

Guidelines for Authorship

In seeking the definition of authorship, what is the test for determining the difference between "earned authorship" and "honorary authorship?" Scientists may hold the former to be right and the latter wrong, but there is certainly a continuum between the two. Making decisions along the continuum is difficult when arguments persist over the definitions of the endpoints—those that are unqualified as acceptable or unacceptable. Considerable agreement exists on what is unacceptable. However, there can be great differences of opinion on what earns someone the right to authorship. Although some journals have provided guidance on defining authorship and its responsibilities, the language includes sweeping statements that provide much latitude for interpretation. Such broad-based guidance is of limited value to the novice writer or trainee.

Definitive answers to questions about authorship and its responsibilities must come from the scientific community itself. In recent years attempts at solutions are coming from the institutions in which scientists practice. Some institutions now publish guidelines on the meaning and definition of authorship. Additionally, there is an increasing related literature that comprises books, editorials, and special articles. A sampling of these kinds of writings, some of which include institutional guidelines, is given in the references section of this chapter.

Authors need to understand and abide by the guidelines of their institutions, if such guidelines exist. If not, the topics covered here should provide a general substrate for thinking about authorship. Discussions among and between trainees, mentors, and colleagues will also clarify the issues and facilitate an understanding of an appreciation for the nuances of authorship.

The following sections outline material collected from various guidelines and deal exclusively with coauthored manuscripts.

The senior author

A familiar term is that of *senior author* (sometimes called *primary author*). Guidelines often define this person as the principal investigator, leader of the group, or laboratory director. If the byline of a paper lists a faculty mentor along with two of her predoctoral trainees and one postdoctoral trainee, then the mentor is the senior author.

The senior author may or may not be the first author listed on the byline. In general, most agree that the first author is defined as having played a major role in generating the data, interpreting the results, and writing the first draft of the manuscript. In many cases, however, the first author and the senior author are different people. When this is so, it is customary for the senior author's name to be last in the byline. Sometimes papers are authored by more than one person of senior status. Most of the time it is still possible to define one of the two as the senior author of the paper, based on their respective contributions as well as the contributing roles of the other coauthors (e.g., in which senior author's lab was the work done). It is sometimes possible for senior authorship to be shared; this designation and the position of the names of the senior authors on the byline should be decided by mutual consent.

Responsibilities of the senior author

Guidelines often vest senior authors with overarching responsibilities. What follows is an amalgamation of the typical responsibilities listed in several documents from universities and research institutions.

The senior author (and first author if different) decides on who else will be listed as coauthors. General criteria for making these decisions are discussed below. The senior author is responsible for notifying all coauthors of this decision and for facilitating discussion and determining the order of appearance of the coauthors' names on the byline.

The senior author (with the help of the first author and sometimes other coauthors) decides as well on the names of people to be listed in the acknowledgments section. The senior author should notify individuals who are to be acknowledged. He or she is also responsible for listing in the acknowledgments all sources of financial support for the work. In short, the senior author is responsible for appropriately acknowledging all variety of contributions to the work reported in the paper.

Senior authors review all data contained in the paper and, in doing so, assume responsibility for the validity of the entire body of work. This assertion, which is commonly being written into institutional guidelines, can present problems when specialized work reported in the paper falls outside the senior author's area of expertise. Here, the senior author should gain a reasonable understanding and verification of the data from the appropriate coauthor. This problem, however, persists as interdisciplinary research proliferates and researchers from highly technical and specialized fields collaborate and copublish their results. Nonetheless, current guidelines are very specific on this point: the senior author must "understand the general principles of all work included in the paper."

The senior author has an additional responsibility to facilitate communication among coauthors during the preparation of the manuscript. This can mean reviewing raw data and discussing new ideas for additional work. It certainly means reaching agreement on the part of all coauthors as to interpretation of results and conclusions. He or she should also be able to describe the role and contributions of all coauthors in the work. Some institutions require that this be done in writing, with the documentation being retained in appropriate departmental files. Some institutions require a signed document from coauthors indicating their approval of the manuscript and their permission to submit it for publication. In fact, there are journals that require that the letter covering the submitted manuscript indicate essentially the same thing; the letter must be signed by every coauthor.

The senior author ensures that the logistics of manuscript submission are properly followed. This would include such things as manuscript format (and related material) and local editorial review where required as well as all dealings with the publisher. Matters associated with the publisher might include things like correspondence, execution of copyright assignments and authorship agreement forms, and, where appropriate, financial arrangements such as page charges and reprint costs. The senior author should establish a policy regarding distribution of reprints of the paper, including the provision of a reasonable number of reprints to all coauthors.

The senior author coordinates and oversees the responses to the peer reviewer's comments if the manuscript has to be revised. He or she should involve the coauthors in this process as appropriate, and seek their approval before submitting the revised manuscript. Once the paper is published, the senior author is responsible for acting on and honoring requests to share materials from the research, as well as for coordinating and making responses to general inquiries or challenges about the work. He or she also assumes responsibility for handling the publication of corrections, errata, or retractions, including coordinating preparation of such items by agreement of all coauthors. Finally, the senior author has responsibility for the appropriate retention and storage of all data used to prepare the manuscript.

The first author
This is the author whose name appears first on the byline of the paper. This person may also be called the principal author (although this can be a confusing term since the senior author is usually a principal investigator). As mentioned earlier, the first author is the person who participated significantly in the work by: (1) doing experiments and collecting the data, (2) interpreting the results, and (3) writing the first draft of the manuscript.

The submitting author
This term is occasionally used to describe the person who sees the manuscript through the submission process: letter writing, coordinating responses to the editor, responding to peer review comments, etc. Sometimes this person is called the corresponding author. This is usually the senior author, but it can be the first author. For example, a mentor (senior author) may want his postdoctoral (first author) to gain experience in dealing with the peer review process. It should be remembered that when this happens certain related responsibilities discussed previously would fall on this author. Many publishers identify

the submitting author on the first page of the published article. Thus, the responsibilities of the senior author with respect to correspondence after publication would lie with the submitting (or corresponding) author when this happens. Where the submitting author and senior author are not the same person, there should be an advanced understanding of how follow-up correspondence related to the manuscript will be handled (e.g., requests for biologic materials, etc.).

Other coauthors

Coauthors whose names appear between the first and last authors on the byline are usually decided upon by the senior author and the first author. The order of these coauthors can be based on the importance of their contributions to the work in descending order from the first author. Decisions on authorship need to be made before the paper is written. It may be appropriate to change the order of the authors as the work and manuscript preparation progress. The senior and first authors should guide any process to revise author order, but such decisions should involve all coauthors.

What counts toward authorship?

Authorship encompasses two fundamental principles: contribution and responsibility. An author must make a significant intellectual or practical contribution to the work reported in the paper. With such authorship goes the responsibility for the contents of the paper. By keeping such concepts simple, the qualitative and quantitative aspects of these contributions and the precise nature of the responsibilities are left open to interpretation. This flexibility is valued by many in the scientific community. Nonetheless, the articulation of authorship contributions and responsibilities by institutions provides clarity that aids both the seasoned and the novice author.

The meaning of "authorship" has been defined in a variety of ways. Significant contributions are frequently described as things that have an effect on the "direction, scope, or depth of the research." They can also include "conceptualization, design, execution, and/or interpretation of the research." The development of necessary methodologies and data analysis essential to the conclusions of the project are also sometimes listed as contributions which justify authorship. Sometimes the language gets specific and contributions to the project are linked to having a "clear understanding of its goals." This leads us to the issue of responsibility.

Responsibility has been linked to authorship as the need "to take responsibility for the defense of the study should the need arise" or "to present and defend the work in context at a scientific meeting." The challenge of coauthor responsibility (where contributions are often disparate) can create exceptions when "one author has carried out a unique, sophisticated study or analysis." In other words, it can be argued that in certain collaborative studies, it may not be possible for every author to be able to rigorously present and defend all aspects of the work.

What doesn't count

In many of the guidelines, naming the things that don't merit authorship has been as helpful as naming those that do. Just providing funding for the work, or status as a group or unit leader, does not alone justify authorship. Neither does providing only lab space or the use of instrumentation. Finally, doing routine technical work on the project, providing services or materials for a fee, or merely editing a manuscript is not sufficient justification for authorship.

Peer Review

Many scientists get called on to review manuscripts. This generally happens in two ways. First, scientists may be appointed as members of editorial boards of scientific journals, in which case their duties as reviewers are formalized. Editorial board members regularly get papers to review and their names appear in each issue of the journal designated them as "reviewing editors" or as editorial board members, or some equivalent term. Second, scientists get asked to be *ad hoc* reviewers. In this case they receive papers to review from editors and are asked to evaluate them as a courtesy. Usually, *ad hoc* reviewers' names are listed in the last journal issue of the year acknowledging them as reviewers. Many scientific journals in the biomedical and natural sciences rely heavily on the services of *ad hoc* reviewers.

Editorial board members and *ad hoc* reviewers provide a critical service. They prepare written evaluations that help the journal editor decide on the acceptability of the submitted manuscripts. Equally important, their comments usually allow the authors to improve their manuscript if it is not acceptable for publication in its current form. A reviewer's commentary may suggest improvements in writing style, presentation of data, or even additional experiments.

A scientist named to an editorial board is likely to receive from the journal editor or publisher guidelines on how to prepare a review. Over time, the editor may give advice on written reviews and offer suggestions on how to improve them, thus providing ongoing guidance to reviewers.

Ad hoc reviewers are often asked to serve before being mailed a manuscript. Such requests may come by phone, fax, or computer mail. At that time it is a good idea for potential reviewers to check with the editor's office to see if guidelines are available. These are usually brief and can be very helpful; reviewers should secure a copy where possible before beginning a review. A novice reviewer is otherwise likely to have a single frame of reference: reviews previously received on their own manuscripts.

The peer review process for scientific articles has come under scrutiny in recent years, and some have called for radical change or complete abolishment. With that said and accepting peer review as an important element of responsible scientific conduct, we will present the process here in two parts. First an examination will be made of the flow of a manuscript through a typical cycle of peer review. This will be followed by a discussion of the duties and responsibilities of the reviewer.

How Peer Review Usually Works

Typically, peer review begins with submission of a manuscript by mail to an editor or to a central office of the journal publisher. In the latter case the office then assigns the manuscript to an appropriate editor. Typical scientific journals have multiple editors who represent the various subspecialties of the subject matter published in them. The editor then reads the paper (or enough of it) to decide on whom to invite to complete the review. Editors may select editorial board members or *ad hoc* reviewers for this job. Typically a single paper is mailed to two or more peer reviewers (also termed "referees"). Some journals have special forms on which to prepare manuscript reviews, but these frequently merely consist blank space for reviewers to write comments. There can also be a separate form for comments that are intended only for the eyes of the editor. The editor asks for the reviewers to complete their evaluations in a specific period of time (usually less than a month). When the completed reviews are returned to the editor, he or she reads them carefully and then makes one of three decisions: (1) to accept the paper, (2) to reject the paper, or (3) to return the paper to the authors for revision. In all cases the editor sends to the authors a letter indicating his or her decision and its basis. Obviously, in the case of outright acceptance, the letter is brief. However, editors are usually specific in their decision letters when explaining rejection or the need for revision. Such letters reflect the editor's own opinions of the paper in view of the reviewers' comments and recommendations and are accompanied by the verbatim copies of the reviewers' comments. Those sections of the review form that indicate reviewers' specific recommendations ("accept", "reject" or "revise") as well as any comments made in confidence to the editor are not sent to the authors. Editors may and do use comments sent to them separately by reviewers to help in composing their decision letter.

For most scientific journals in the biomedical and natural sciences, the comments of the reviewers are anonymous. However, some journals do reveal reviewer identity to the authors. This can be done as a matter of policy or by encouraging reviewers to sign their written reviews. At least one journal publishes the reviewers' comments along with the corresponding papers.

Authors must consider the reviewers' and editor's comments in revising their papers. They may make changes based on comments they agree with. Alternatively, authors have the right to rebut any and all criticisms of the reviewers. The basis for handling each reviewer's comments must be explained to the editor in a letter that accompanies the revised manuscript. It is then the editor's job to reach a final decision on the paper and to notify the authors.

Being a Peer Reviewer

What to do when the manuscript arrives

There are a number of "housekeeping" chores that reviewers must do when a manuscript is received by mail and it is important (and courteous) to attend to these quickly. First, the reviewer must scan the paper and decide whether he or she is qualified to review it as well as whether he or she can complete the review in the time being allotted by the editor. If the reviewer is uncomfortable with either of these criteria, the manuscript should immediately be sent back to be reassigned. At this time, reviewers should check that they have a complete version of the manuscript. Are all the pages, figures, and tables there? If things are missing or illegible (e.g., photocopies of micrographs instead of originals), the editor or editorial office should be contacted about the missing or needed material.

Reviewers must be comfortable with their ability to impartially review the work. In other words, their review of the paper must not constitute a conflict of interest—real or perceived. Some journals have guidelines for this. As mentioned earlier, typically cited conflicts include papers from investigators at the reviewer's institution, trainees who have recently been in the reviewer's lab, or collaborators of the reviewer at other institutions. Commercial interests also create conflicts. For example, is the paper authored by scientists at a company that pays the reviewer as a consultant or has made a grant or gift to the reviewer's research program? Conflict of interest decisions of this type usually rest with the reviewer. Usually, the information that points to the conflict is known to the reviewer and not the editor and hence he might never become aware of it. The reviewer has to decide whether there is conflict or whether others might perceive specific actions as conflict. A simple rule is, when in doubt, don't review the paper. The reviewer may contact the editor to seek advice on matters of potential conflict. In general, any extensive rationalization for overcoming what might be a perceived conflict is usually a signal to both the reviewer and the editor that a real conflict may exist or may be perceived to exist by others. In such cases, reassignment of the manuscript to another reviewer is necessary.

If a reviewer returns a manuscript for reassignment, it is an accepted courtesy to tell the editor the reason for doing so. It is also customary to suggest the names of potential substitutes. Such assistance is valuable and editors appreciate it.

Philosophy of review
The peer reviewer's task is twofold: (1) to help the editor make a good decision on the acceptability of the paper, and (2) to help the authors communicate their work accurately and effectively. The peer reviewer does not have to be an adversary to do either of these jobs; indeed, in the latter case, he or she should be an advocate for the authors. Guidelines sometimes tell reviewers to take a positive attitude toward the manuscript, and this is good advice. Reviews who are confrontational are distressing to authors and often make things difficult for

all involved. Meaning can get lost in impolite and ill-considered language, and can confuse an editor's attempt to effectively evaluate the reviewer's comments. It can also distract and mislead authors in preparing their rebuttals. Issues can be clouded by offensive language. Authors may "miss the point" and in doing so fail to improve their manuscript. Additionally, time is often wasted as authors feel the need to respond in kind to offensive comments in their rebuttal letters to editors.

Confidentiality

A manuscript sent to a reviewer is a privileged communication and represents confidential information. It should not be copied by any means nor shared with colleagues. Under no circumstances should the reviewer get assistance from colleagues in performing the review without explicit permission of the editor.

A customary policy is that a peer reviewer never contact an author directly about the manuscript under review. This may sound like unnecessary advice, because most journals use anonymous review. However, even if journals allow disclosure of the reviewer's identity to the authors, direct contact between the two during the review process is usually forbidden. The information the reviewer provides on the merit and acceptability of a manuscript is considered by the editor, who makes the final decision. By talking to authors, reviewers may communicate misleading messages that can make the editor's job difficult. Thus, reviewers who need clarification or additional information should always contact the editor and let him or her obtain it.

Commonly used criteria for evaluating merit

The manuscript should contain a clear statement of the problem being studied and it should be put in perspective. Reviewers should evaluate this perspective in the context of appropriate literature citations. In other words, do the authors give appropriate credit to prior work in the field, especially those contributions upon which the present report is built? The originality of the work should be carefully weighed. The reviewer should consider whether the manuscript reports a new discovery as opposed to extending or confirming some previous work.

Experimental techniques and research design should be appropriate to the study. Did the authors use the right tools and techniques to test their hypotheses? Description of methods is very important.

This is the part of scientific communication that allows verification of the work. The description of the materials and methods should be in sufficient detail that other investigators in the field can repeat the work. It is, however, appropriate that some methods be briefly mentioned and then cited in the reference section of the paper. However, it is important that such citations refer to the source where complete methods are described. Papers should not be used as methods citations if they contain incomplete descriptions, or if they refer to yet another paper for the details of some or all of the method.

The reviewer should examine the presentation of data for clarity and effectiveness, keeping in mind several questions. Is data presentation cluttered or confusing? Are figures and photographs clear? What about the organization of the data in tables and figures? Are there too many tables or figures? Can some be deleted? Are data given in tabular form better presented in figures? Should data in tables be combined or single-panel figures be redone as multipanel ones?

Interpretations of the data need to be sound and clearly worded. The discussion of the work should be appropriate: arguments should be logically presented and any speculation should be built on the present work and the existing literature.

The writing in the manuscript should be clear, easy to follow, and grammatically correct. Many guidelines affirm that the peer reviewer's job is not to rewrite the manuscript. However, some comments by the peer reviewer citing examples of writing deficiencies will help the authors when making global revisions. The reviewer should also note whether the authors are adhering to correct scientific nomenclature and abbreviations as specified by the journal.

The reviewer should evaluate the title and abstract after reading the paper. Are they adequate and appropriate? As electronic communications increase, the availability of abstracts is becoming widespread. The abstract has become the "first line" of scientific communication in this medium; therefore, the abstract needs to clearly describe the essence of the problem, how it was attacked, and the outcome of the research.

Writing the review
The actual format for preparing a manuscript review varies from journal to journal. However, it is typical for a review to begin with a paragraph or two that includes a summary of the major findings and

highlights of the paper. If there are overriding considerations, either positive or negative, they should be presented in this narrative. Shortcomings or flaws that have influenced the reviewer's assessment of the paper should be stated in general terms; specific comments can be included later in the review.

Following this narrative, it is customary for the reviewer to list specific, numbered comments. Numbering makes it easier for the authors to respond to the critique and for the editor to make a final decision. Specific comments should offer guidance to the authors on how to improve the work. Problems should be identified and solutions suggested where possible.

Finally, it is customary to not indicate in the narrative or in the specific comments the ultimate recommendation for the paper. Instead, this should be clearly transmitted to the editor. As mentioned earlier, it is commonly done with a specific form, or by a brief note to the editor. There is a reason for this. Rarely do editors merely send a paper to one reviewer; as stated earlier, using two or three experts is the norm. Reviewers can and do disagree about the merits of the same paper. When this occurs, it is the editor's job to sort out the reviews and then write his or her final disposition in a decision letter to the author. It does not help the editor and it frustrates the authors to read two verbatim reviews, one of which explicitly recommends acceptance while the other recommends rejection.

Conclusion

Written communication is an essential part of scientific research. Science can benefit society only insofar as its findings are published and applied. Indeed, biomedical scientists have a moral obligation to share new knowledge in order to advance and improve the health and well-being of humankind. Scientific knowledge is accepted only when the published research results that support it hold up under scrutiny and independent corroboration. The duties and responsibilities of scientific authorship are not to be taken lightly. Historically, many of the decisions about authorship on scientific papers were based on unwritten norms and standards. In recent years, written guidelines for authorship are being promulgated by institutions, societies, and journal publication boards. These provide guidance to authors and they can be especially informative to the novice writer.

Providing peer review of scientific publications is an obligation that is shared by scientists. While peer review must be scholarly and rigorous, it must also be timely, respectful, and courteous. Above all, peer review must be constructive. Peer review plays a vital role in the publication of research findings, although the process is being increasingly challenged. Its workings and effectiveness are likely to be the subjects of continuing debate among scientists for years to come. Nonetheless, the process of peer review is performed under both written and unwritten guidelines. Explicit descriptions of duties and responsibilities of peer reviewers are now frequently published by scientific journals. In part, these aim to foster consistency and integrity in the process.

Case Studies

4.1 You are a member of a large scientific society that publishes several peer-reviewed journals. The publications board of this society has proposed a new rule that is being voted upon by the entire society. The rule states: "Any manuscript submitted for publication in a journal of the society which lists more than 4 (four) authors must be accompanied by a letter from the corresponding author stating the respective contributions of each and every listed author on the manuscript." How will you vote? Why? Discuss your perception of the proposed rule, including any modifications you'd like to see made to it.

4.2 An investigator has published a brief description of a bacterial mutant strain (including data on a biochemical assay of its phenotype) as a full-length paper in a peer-reviewed journal. She is contacted by a colleague who requests the mutant strain. The colleague clearly describes his intended use for the mutant in studies which are presently ongoing in his laboratory. The author of the manuscript refuses to release the strain. She cites that it was only described in a preliminary way in the paper. Moreover, she indicates that another major manuscript is in preparation in which the particular mutant will be the central focus of the report. She says she will be happy to release the mutant after the second manuscript has been accepted for publication. Is the investigator justified in her actions? Why or why not?

4.3 An investigator prepares a manuscript for submission to a prestigious journal in cell biology. A colleague of his in a separate department at the same institution is a member of the journal's editorial board. The investigator submits the manuscript for consideration by the journal to his institutional colleague. They briefly discuss conflict of interest implications of this action but decide that because the manuscript will be reviewed by at least two outside referees, it can be appropriately handled by the editor without a perceived conflict of interest. Do you agree or disagree with this decision? Why or why not?

4.4 A member of an NIH study section is in the process of reviewing several grants assigned to her in connection with an upcoming meeting of the study section. During this process, she receives by mail a manuscript from a journal editor and is asked to review it as an *ad hoc* reviewer. The author of the manuscript turns out to be the principal investigator of one of the grants the study section member is currently reviewing. Indeed, the manuscript in question has been submitted as an appendix to the grant application. The study section member elects to review the manuscript sent to her by the journal editor. Comment on the appropriateness of her decision to review the paper.

4.5 A faculty member receives a manuscript for *ad hoc* review from the editor of a scientific journal. He gives the manuscript to a senior postdoctoral associate in his group and asks her to read the manuscript and prepare some written comments on it. One week later, she provides one page of handwritten comments to the faculty member and they briefly discuss the manuscript. The faculty member then prepares a written review which is submitted to the editor of the scientific journal. A few weeks later, the faculty member learns that the postdoctoral associate made photocopies of the entire literature citation section of the manuscript because it contained "some useful references." The faculty member proceeds to reprimand the postdoctoral associate, telling her that no part of a manuscript received for review should be copied. Comment on the behavior of both the faculty member and the postdoctoral associate in this scenario.

4.6 A graduate student in a cell biology department has purified two recombinant proteins as part of his dissertation research. These proteins differ only in a few key amino acid positions. Based on standard available biochemical data, the student believes the proteins are virtually identical. In discussions with a graduate student from the biochemistry department, the cell biology student concludes that it would be reasonable to compare these two purified proteins by circular dichroism. The graduate student in biochemistry offers to collaborate on the project by analyzing the two proteins by this technique and presenting the data to the cell biology student. The faculty advisor of the biochemistry student is told of this and he proceeds to tell the advisor of the cell biology student that he expects this will be a fruitful collaboration which should result in a coauthored publication. He argues that his rationale for this is based on his student's intellectual contribution in presenting the data and operating highly technical instrumentation and on his own intellectual and financial support of the circular dichroism instrument facility. The advisor of the cell biology student is strongly opposed to a coauthored paper, arguing that the biochemistry student's contribution is largely technical and does not merit coauthorship. He suggests that the biochemistry graduate student's name be placed in the acknowledgment section of any paper that comes from this work and that any of his mentor's grants used to support the circular dichroism facility be cited in the acknowledgments as well. Discuss the relevant issues of authorship in this case. Are there facts which are not presented that might sway you one way or the other in terms of resolving the differences between the two mentors? What would be some examples of such facts?

4.7 A faculty investigator develops a DNA probe as a "side project" working under NIH grant funding. Although not immediately applicable, this DNA has potential in the diagnosis of a latent viral disease in humans. She publishes her results in a peer-reviewed scientific journal. Following the appearance of this work, the faculty investigator is called by a director of research of a large U.S. pharmaceutical firm. The research director requests a plasmid carrying the probe sequence for use in his company's research. The research director assures the faculty investigator that the company has no intent of commercializing the DNA probe. The investigator refuses to comply with the request for the DNA probe, claiming that the potential for commercialization is always present in the research environment of a for-profit company. The director of research counters with the fact that the faculty investigator has published her results and must release the material under the standards of publication set by the peer-reviewed journal. What are the intellectual property and data ownership considerations that surround this issue? Can it be resolved? How?

4.8 A colleague has come to you for advice regarding a recently published paper which contains data similar to results he published approximately six months previously. Your colleague is upset because the paper reaches the same conclusions as his work using somewhat similar approaches, yet the authors fail to cite his work. Although he personally does not know any of the authors on the paper, your colleague can't imagine that they have not seen his previously published work. Both his paper and the new manuscript have appeared in different but comparable journals of the discipline. He is very upset about this matter and seeks your advice on what, if anything, he can and should do. What do you tell him?

4.9 A new postdoctoral is recruited to a laboratory where research is centered on the cell biology of a specific mammalian cell type. The postdoctoral's training has been in eucaryotic gene cloning and molecular genetics; no such technology is available in this laboratory or the department. The new postdoctoral completely trains a senior-level graduate student working in the group. The student proceeds to build a cDNA library of the cell type in question and isolates by molecular cloning a gene for a membrane protein. Several months later a manuscript describing this work is prepared for submission. The principal investigator (PI) of the laboratory and student are listed as coauthors. The postdoctoral is listed in the acknowledgment section of the paper. The postdoctoral is upset with this disposition and confronts the principal investigator. The PI indicates that she has strict rules about authorship and that the postdoctoral's contribution was a technical one which does not merit qualification for authorship. The PI quotes from several different standards-of-conduct documents indicating that authorship must be strictly based on intellectual and conceptual contributions to the work being prepared for publication. Technical assistance, no matter how complex or broad in scope, is not grounds for authorship. Comment on this situation.

4.10 You are an editor of a journal. Manuscript reviews are handled in confidence and *ad hoc* reviewers are always sent guidelines regarding confidentiality. They include statements that restrict the divulging of manuscript contents to anyone, or using results reported in the paper to advance one's own research. You carefully check manuscripts before sending them out for review to ensure that they are complete with respect to text pages, tables, figures, etc. A stapled copy of a manuscript is sent out to an *ad hoc* reviewer (with confidentiality guidelines). Two weeks later the paper is returned with a negative review, recommending rejection of the paper on the grounds of its results being too preliminary (although potentially exciting). You happen to notice that the manuscript has had the original staple removed and apparently has been restapled. This prompts you to examine the entire paper, upon which you discover the text page 9 is missing but there are duplicate page 10s. Based on this, you suspect that the reviewer has photocopied the manuscript and has retained a copy. What, if anything, do you do as editor? Would any of your proposed actions differ if the review had been positive, recommending acceptance of the paper?

4.11 You are editor-in-chief of a prestigious cell biology journal. About a year ago you personally handled and accepted an important manuscript (from Dr. Barbara Smith) which described a novel tumor cell line. This cell line derives from an unusual rodent liver tumor, grows rapidly *in vivo,* and produces several new membrane proteins. You recently read a paper from another research group (Dr. Jeffrey Wilson) that reports the cloning and characterization of one of these novel membrane protein genes. Shortly after the appearance of the Wilson group's paper, you receive a phone call from Dr. Smith. She is upset and claims Dr. Wilson has acted unethically. She goes on to say that Dr. Wilson requested the cell line from her, explaining that his reason for wanting it was to explore its genome for standard and novel retrovirus genes. The cell line specifically was released to Dr. Wilson with that understanding, agreed to by both parties in writing. Dr. Smith is upset because her group had been working on the cloning of the genes specifying the novel membrane proteins; now they have been partially "scooped" by Dr. Wilson. She accuses Dr. Wilson of obtaining the cell line under false pretenses. Dr. Smith asks your advice on what to do. She specifically requests that you pursue this as editor-in-chief of the journal, claiming that the behavior violates common publication ethics. What advice do you provide? What, if any, are your responsibilities as editor-in-chief? What, if any, actions do you take as editor-in-chief? Consult the "publication policies" documents from one or more appropriate journals to assist you in your deliberations and decision.

4.12 You are editor-in-chief of a major scientific journal. You receive a call from Dr. Martha Green, who indicates that she has discovered that a member of your editorial board has received a paper listing her name (along with three other individuals) as an author. Dr. Green indicates that, although one member of her research team performed some experiments in his laboratory during a summer sabbatical,

Green herself was not involved in the writing of the research paper nor was she sent a copy of the manuscript prior to its submission. The scientific journal of which you are the editor-in-chief has very stringent regulations on defining authorship and has as its explicit policy that manuscripts be submitted with the full knowledge and full approval of all individuals listed as authors. Dr. Green is very uncomfortable with what has happened and asks your advice on how to proceed. What advice do you provide? What, if any, action do you take with regard to this manuscript? The timing of events is such that the paper was submitted approximately one month ago. This means that your editorial board member has undoubtedly sent the manuscript out to at least two expert reviewers in the field.

REFERENCES

1. **American Chemical Society.** 1994. Ethical guidelines to publication of chemical research. *Acc. Chem. Res.* **27:**179–181.
2. **Bailar, J., M. Angell, S. Boots, E. Myers, N. Palmer, M. Shipley, and P. Woolf.** 1990. *Ethics and Policy in Scientific Publication.* Editorial Policy Committee, Council of Biology Editors, Bethesda, MD.
3. **Booth, V.** 1993. *Communicating in Science,* 2nd ed. Cambridge University Press, New York.
4. **Day, R. A.** 1994. *How to Write and Publish a Scientific Paper,* 4th ed. Oryx Press, Phoenix, AZ.
5. **MacDermott, R. P.** 1991. Fraudulent research in science: the responsibility of the peer reviewer. *Cancer Invest.* **9:**703–705.
6. **National Academy of Sciences.** 1993. *Responsible Science,* Vol. II: *Ensuring the Integrity of the Research Process.* National Academy Press, Washington, D.C. (This volume contains guidelines on responsible conduct, including criteria for authorship, used at several institutions.)
7. **Tipton, C. M.** 1991. Publishing in peer-reviewed journals—fundamentals for the new investigator. *Physiologist* **34:**275–279.
8. **Walton, S.** 1987. Coauthorship responsibility issue under study. *Scientist* **1:** 1, 8. (Describes policy adopted by one institution.)
9. **Waser, N. M., M. V. Price, and R. K. Grosberg.** 1992. Writing an effective manuscript review. *BioScience* **42:**621–623.

5 | Use of Animals in Biomedical Experimentation

Bruce A. Fuchs

Introduction

A consensus challenged

Animal experimentation has been an important research tool for more than 100 years. At the dawn of the 19th century, scientific medicine was beginning to challenge medical traditions more than a thousand years old. Physiological research involving animals was one of the key technologies which spurred this transition and led to an understanding of bodily functions and the physical basis of disease. However, the new approach was resisted by traditionalists who employed as one of their foremost criticisms the cruel nature of animal research. Present-day scientists should not delude themselves; early animal experiments could be exceedingly brutal. Fully conscious dogs were nailed to boards by their four paws, prior to being cut open, so that the beating of a heart might be observed. While the advent of anesthesia in the mid-1800s addressed some concerns, it by no means ended the debate over the fundamental morality of animal research. Numerous groups formed in the late 1800s to challenge the existing social order with regard to animals. These "antivivisectionists" were the antecedents of the contemporary "animal rights" movement.

In 1975 Peter Singer, an Australian philosopher, published the book *Animal Liberation* (46), which many credit as comprising the seminal event in the rebirth of modern antivivisectionism. Over the past 15 years, animal rights activists have assiduously set about achieving their ultimate goal—the abolition of the use of animals for biomedical research, food, clothing, and entertainment. The most extreme activists question even the morality of pet ownership. The animal rights movement is viewed by many scientists as a threat to scientific progress and, ultimately, to the health and well-being of humankind. Nevertheless, the majority of scientists have not actively participated in the debate by responding to the charges of the animal rights activists at the local level, preferring instead to allow a defense to be mounted by national scientific organizations. This is arguably a serious mistake. The animal rights organizations have been extraordinarily successful in carrying their message to the general public. While the majority of the population still expresses support for the use of animals in biomedical research, the efforts of animal rights activists have clearly eroded this support, especially among young people. Additionally, the animal rights movement has sought to link its agenda with that of other popular causes, such as environmentalism, saying in essence, "If you care about our environment you must support animal rights."

It is important that individual scientists take the time to become better educated about the moral and political controversies which surround the use of animals in biomedical research. Scientists often have a tendency to dismiss the animal rights philosophy as irrational. Yet the movement's leading philosophers, people like Peter Singer and Tom Regan, are respected scholars who present eloquently argued, and intensely rational, cases for their belief in animal "rights." Inadequately prepared scientists can embarrass themselves and the larger scientific community in trying to debate some of the articulate, well-prepared leaders of the animal rights community. One will not catch these individuals in trivial moral blunders—they do not eat meat, wear leather shoes, or frequent the circus. Many of them struggle to live an ethically consistent (and difficult to maintain) lifestyle because of the moral status which they ascribe to animals. The fact that scientists are often unfamiliar with the ethical theories of the leading animal rights philosophers is bound to reduce their effectiveness in any public debate of the issues.

Scientists occasionally have a tendency to dismiss all animal rights activists as the members of a "lunatic fringe." This view is untenable. The vast majority of people in attendance at animal rights meetings are not lunatics, but rather people just like our neighbors. It is important to realize that most of the people at such meetings are not fervent animal rights activists. They continue to eat meat, value the benefits of medical research, and own pets, no matter what their leadership might have to say about these practices. These people are, however, extremely concerned about how the animals used in biomedical research are being treated. And unfortunately, their major source of information is often the animal rights groups themselves. Because of this they are often inherently distrustful of the scientific establishment. It is not likely that any impersonal scientific organization is going to be able to quiet their fears without the help of large numbers of individual scientists explaining to their own neighbors exactly how they do biomedical research.

"Rights" for animals?

While most scientists would probably not claim that animals have rights, it is important to realize that we nevertheless act as though animals do have something *like* rights. It is worth spending a moment to consider why most working scientists support the use of animals in biomedical research, and are also concerned that such research be conducted humanely. Likewise, while fairly large percentages of the general public (especially young people) express support for the concept of animals rights, they simultaneously eat animals and support the use of animals in biomedical research. Therefore, while it is apparent that nearly all of us perceive animals to be objects of moral concern, the exact nature and extent of our moral obligations are not entirely clear.

If asked to describe the difference between a test tube and a mouse, none of you would have any problem in doing so. Precisely how you choose to reply might well depend on whether you have been trained in biology, chemistry, genetics, etc. However, it seems likely that your initial answer would focus around the most compelling distinction between the test tube and the mouse—the fact that the mouse is a living creature. Now let's suppose that someone enters your laboratory with a hammer and smashes one of your test tubes. Clearly it would be wrong for them to do so. They would have intentionally, and senselessly, destroyed your property. To be sure, in these days of disposable culture tubes, the actual loss to you would be a small one. But now let us change the scenario and suppose that instead of destroying one of your test tubes, the person enters your laboratory to smash one of your mice. This act, too, would be wrong. But is it wrong for precisely the same reasons as the previous destruction of the test tube? The person has once again destroyed your property, and it is also true that the mouse is undoubtedly worth more in purely monetary terms. But is this the full measure of the difference between these acts? Few of us would equate the senseless destruction of a whole shelf pack of test tubes (to equalize the monetary value) with that of a single laboratory mouse.

It is important to understand that ownership of property is not the key issue. What if, instead of using the hammer to smash your mouse, the person in question used it to smash one of their own? How many would feel significantly better about the event? So what is the fundamental difference in the destruction of these two objects? Is it only the fact that the mouse is alive while the test tube is not? Then let's suppose that it is not a test tube that is about to be destroyed, but rather a tissue culture flask full of living cells. Clearly, the senseless destruction of a mouse is more troubling than that of a flask of cells. Therefore it is not the mere fact that the mouse is alive that we are responding to—it must be something else.

Moral judgments
At some level, many scientists are abolitionists. That is, if we were able to acquire the information needed to adequately answer compelling research questions without the use of animals, who among us would not gladly do so? Nevertheless, one of the best methods we have developed to advance biomedical knowledge involves the use of animals which, unlike the test tube, have interests. They have interests in obtaining sufficient food, in remaining free from pain, in reproducing themselves, and perhaps in living a normal life span. Experiments can frustrate the interests of laboratory animals, and most scientists recognize this both in their concern for the humane treatment of animals and in their belief that research should be directed at important problems. The fact that animals have interests does not necessarily mean that we should never use them in biomedical experiments; however, it does mean that any such use should be preceded by a moral judgment. Do the benefits derived from biomedical research being considered offset the associated moral costs?

Animal rights groups are challenging the existing societal consensus on many questions involving animals. In the next decade, public policy decisions concerning animals are likely to be made at a rate unparalleled since the first wave of antivivisectionist activity began more than 100 years ago. These decisions will be made whether or not scientists choose to participate in the ongoing public debates over the issues.

The Underlying Philosophical Issues

It is unfortunate that many working in the biomedical sciences have had little formal introduction to the field of ethics, as they may as a consequence have little appreciation for its power as a discipline. Occasionally those working in the sciences are suspicious that "soft" disciplines such as moral philosophy lack the type of academic rigor displayed by their own fields. It is not uncommon for scientists to criticize animal rights activists for being excessively emotional and insufficiently rational. Yet such a charge cannot be appropriately leveled at the principal philosophers of the animal rights movement, including Peter Singer and Tom Regan. These individuals are respected scholars who present rational, not emotional, arguments in favor of granting animals far more moral weight than society presently allows them. We will consider the differing philosophical traditions from which each of these philosophers is attempting to persuade our society that many of its traditional uses of animals are immoral.

What are ethics?

Some people believe that ethical opinions are mere preferences akin to expressing a taste for a flavor of ice cream, or type of music. For these people there is little basis (or reason) for differentiating among ethical positions. However, there are few philosophers who would seriously argue for such a "strongly subjective" view of ethics. We make rational decisions about our ethical positions in a way we do not about ice cream. If a friend expresses a preference for strawberry none of us would feel compelled to argue the merits of chocolate. This would not be the case for a friend expressing an intent to commit murder. However, ethics are also not "strongly objective" in the manner of many scientific principles. Scientists anywhere around the world, or at any time throughout history, who seek to measure the density of pure gold will find, within the error of their instruments, the same result. Yet there is no comparable experiment which we could perform to assess the morality of a practice, such as polygamy, which is acceptable in some cultures and taboo in others. Ethics fall in between these extreme positions. They are neither matters of taste nor immutable physical constants which can be objectively determined irrespective of time and culture. Then what are ethics? Side-stepping this difficult question, ethics as a discipline is a branch of philosophy which is concerned with morality. Ethics is usually sub-divided into two areas known as normative ethics and metaethics. Normative ethics seeks to establish which behavior is morally right or wrong; that is, it seeks to establish norms for our behavior. Normative ethics is persuasive in that it attempts to set out a moral theory which can be used to determine which views are acceptable and ought to be adopted. This differs from metaethics, which concerns itself with an analysis of fundamental moral concepts, for example, concepts of right and wrong, or of duty. We will not discuss metaethics, but will focus instead on some of the normative ethical theories which attempt to persuade us to radically redefine our behavior toward animals.

While not all philosophers advance identical ethical theories, this fact should not be attributed to any inherent weakness in the discipline. It is not at all uncommon for two biomedical scientists to disagree on the implications of a certain data set. It is quite possible that the two scientists are approaching the problem with different hypotheses in mind. Likewise, given an ethical dilemma, one will often find ethicists who reach differing conclusions as to the best course of action. The difference of opinion may be attributable to the fact that each ethicist has tried to solve the dilemma by using a different normative ethical theory. Alternatively, they may have each used a similar ethical theory and yet differed greatly in the amount of weight each ascribed to the various components of the problem. In addition, there can be disagreements over the empirical facts of a case (for example, in whether an animal feels pain during a given procedure). The point is that moral problem solving, like biological problem solving, is an extremely complex process, and we should not be surprised to find that different people do not always arrive at the same conclusion.

However, it is equally important to realize that while many ethical dilemmas may not have a single "right" answer, there are answers which are clearly wrong. Who would seriously argue that ethical decisions should be made by tossing a coin, or that abortions should be considered moral on Mondays and immoral on Tuesdays? Ethical positions can be evaluated and compared using techniques which are not entirely foreign to those in the sciences. Ethical theories as well can be evaluated on the basis of their rationality, their consistency, and even their usefulness.

While the evaluation of competing ethical theories is a difficult task, there are areas of general agreement where we might begin (31). Ethical theories, like any other, are expected to be internally consistent. No theory should be allowed to contradict itself. Similarly, theories which are unclear or incomplete are clearly less valuable than theories which do not suffer from these flaws. Simplicity could also be considered an advantage. If all else were equal, it would be preferable to employ a simple theory over one which is complex or difficult to apply. We should also require that an ethical theory provide us with assistance in those dilemmas where intuition fails to provide us with a clear answer. Most real-life ethical dilemmas are considered as such precisely because compelling moral arguments can be made in support of each side of the issue. These types of situations are those in which we most require the guidance of a moral theory. Additionally, ethical theories should generally agree with our sense of moral intuition. Who would wish to adopt an ethic which, although consistent, complete, and simple, advocated murder for profit? However, it is more difficult to decide about a theory which runs counter to our moral intuition in an area less clear-cut than murder. What should we think of a theory which runs counter to our intuition in a number of minor areas? This is where the evaluation process becomes extremely difficult (12). How are we to decide whether it is the theory or our intuition which is out of line? We may decide that if a theory is rational, is well designed, and gives answers which correspond to our moral intuition on a large range of issues, then in a particular instance it is our intuition which should be altered.

We in the natural sciences have something of an advantage over moral philosophers. Usually, we can design an experiment to discern which of two competing hypotheses is most correct. Philosophers do not have the luxury of performing an experiment and letting the data decide between the competing theories. However, ethicists do continually subject their own philosophies, and those of their colleagues, to "thought experiments" involving real or hypothetical ethical dilemmas. This process involves using a particular ethical theory to perform the moral calculus needed to answer a problem. It is sometimes found that the rigorous application of an ethical theory will lead to an outcome which is unacceptable, either to the philosopher or to the larger society. The philosopher may then decide to modify the theory in hopes of increasing its acceptability, or may choose to stick with the theory and instead suggest that it is society itself which ought to be modified.

Utilitarianism

Ethical theories are generally divided into two major categories. The first of these is called either *teleological* or *consequentialist,* and the second is referred to as *deontological.* Teleological theories focus exclusively on the consequences of an action in order to determine the morality of that action. Thus to determine if a particular act is moral or immoral, one determines whether the consequences of that act are considered to be good or bad. Those theories which do not exclusively evaluate the consequences of an act to determine its morality are called deontological theories and will be considered in the next section. The best-known example of a teleological theory is utilitarianism. Jeremy Bentham (1748–1832) was the first person to articulate the theory under that name and John Stuart Mill (1806–1873) was also influential in its development. Utilitarianism acknowledges the fact that many acts do not produce purely good consequences or purely bad consequences, but some combination of the two. In order to decide whether a particular act is moral, a person must sum up all of the consequences, both good and bad, in order to assess the net outcome. Moral actions are those which cause the best balance of good versus bad consequences.

In addition, utilitarianism requires a person to consider the interests of everyone. It is not permissible to merely consider what is best for you personally. Suppose that you are considering lying about the results of an experiment which you have performed. You reason that lying about the experiment will greatly increase the chance of your paper being accepted by a prestigious journal. This will, in turn, enhance your career, your salary, your family's security, etc. However, utilitarianism requires that you also consider the impact of your decision to lie on other people. You must consider the fact that the people who read your paper and are misled by its fabricated results may be harmed by your decision. Some of these people may decide to initiate a new series of experiments, or alternatively, to cease a line of investigation based on your fabricated data. If your research has direct clinical relevance, it is possible that patients may be directly injured or killed by your deceit. If you are caught in your lie, still more harm will accrue both to you directly and to the public's confidence in science. If you consider the cumulative negative impact of your lying on everyone, and not just the positive benefits which you are seeking, it will become apparent that the net outcome is a bad one. According to utilitarian theory, this act of deceit is immoral and you ought not carry it out. Now let's imagine a very different situation. A mentally insane relative of one of your colleagues has escaped and shows up at the lab where you both work. Waving a scalpel and screaming that he wants to kill your friend for "ruining his life," he asks you to tell him where she is working. Although you know exactly where she is, what should you do? After performing the same type of utilitarian calculus as above, it is clear that you should lie to the escaped patient. The net of good and bad consequences which will flow out of this particular act of deceit is markedly different from the scenario described above. Thus we find in utilitarianism ethical decisions which change as circumstances change. An act which is deemed immoral under one set of circumstances can become morally obligatory under another. But exactly what are we to consider when we try to evaluate good and bad consequences? According to Mill, the only good is happiness and the only bad is unhappiness. Bentham thought that pleasure was the only good and that pain was the only bad. These terms are defined somewhat more broadly than you might imagine. Pleasure includes such things as satisfaction of desires, attainment of goals, and enjoyment, while pain includes, in addition to physical discomfort, things such as the frustration of one's goals or desires.

Utilitarianism, like all other ethical theories, has its critics. One criticism is that it is excessively burdensome to employ. Utilitarianism requires that we *all* evaluate how *each* of our actions will affect *everyone*. How is it possible to actually do this? How is it possible to predict the consequences of even a fairly simple action on *everyone*? If we are required to do this for each of our actions, how will we be able to get anything accomplished? The advice to use our "common sense" does not seem to be very helpful. Another criticism of utilitarianism is that it would appear to condone, or even mandate, some actions which most of us would find horrendous. Suppose we find a patient who has a lymphoma which is producing a substance of tremendous use in the treatment of AIDS. However, the patient is totally uncooperative, refusing to either accept treatment for his illness or allow samples of his cells to be taken for research purposes. Utilitarianism might allow us to kill this person and divide his cells among the interested research labs. While one person would die, many AIDS patients would live. Utilitarianism is potentially at odds with our concepts of individual human rights.

Singer's utilitarianism and animal "rights"

Peter Singer is the Australian moral philosopher whose book *Animal Liberation* is credited with the modern revival of the animal rights movement when it was first published in 1975 (46). There is a small irony in this because Singer, like Bentham before him, does not believe in the philosophical concept of rights. Although Singer uses the term "rights," he does not consider it to have philosophical meaning, but instead to be a "convenient political shorthand" (45). Singer echoes Bentham's assertion that the key moral question related to animals is not whether they can reason, but whether they suffer. For Singer sentience, the ability to feel pleasure or pain, is the key characteristic required for admittance into the moral universe. Singer concludes that many animals can suffer from physical pain, deprivation, or loneliness, while he also fully acknowledges that humans can suffer in ways that animals cannot (e.g., the fear of a future catastrophe.) Singer, again drawing from Bentham, proposes that a principle of equality requires that we give equal consideration to the suffering of individuals, regardless of their species. Failure to do so amounts to *speciesism*, an offense which Singer finds analogous to racism or sexism (43,46). It is important to realize that Singer is not claiming that there are no relevant moral differences between humans and animals. Human children have an interest in learning to read. Therefore, it would be immoral for us to raise a child and intentionally prevent him or her from acquiring this skill. Clearly, such disapprobation is meaningless for animals who have no interest (or capability) in reading. Nevertheless, Singer argues that both animals and humans have an equal interest in being free from torment. Because of this, he maintains that it is just as wrong to torture an animal as it is a human being. But once again, this does not mean that Singer believes that all lives are of equal moral worth. He plainly states that if one is required to decide between the life of a human being and the life of a nonhuman animal, then one should choose to save the life of the human (45). Singer can envision circumstances which might alter this decision. If the life of a normal animal is placed in the balance with that of a severely impaired human, the normal decision might be reversed and the life of the animal saved.

Thus, Singer does not say it is never appropriate to use animals in scientific research. As a utilitarian, he *must* support such use if the benefits obtained outweigh the harm done. But Singer places an enormous barrier in the way of such research, one he believes will forbid essentially all of it. Since pain in animals and humans is viewed as exacting an equivalent moral cost, no animal experiment should be conducted unless it would also be permitted on a human.

> We have seen that experimenters reveal a bias in favor of their own species whenever they carry out experiments on nonhumans for purposes that they would not think justified them in using human beings, even brain damaged ones. This principle gives us a guide toward an answer to our question. Since a speciesist bias, like a racist bias, is unjustifiable, an experiment cannot be justifiable unless the experiment is so important that the use of a brain-damaged human would also be justifiable. (44)

It is clear that Singer does not believe that very much animal research would be able to overcome this obstacle. It is also clear that he does not believe this loss to be a serious one. He believes that "animal experimentation has made at best a very small contribution to our increased lifespan" (44). For Singer the benefits of animal research (or of meat eating) are not worth the moral costs.

Singer's philosophy has been criticized by fellow utilitarian R. G. Frey of Bowling Green State University (19,20). Frey defends the use of animals in medical research, using essentially the same utilitarian ethic as does Singer! In some of their writings, it is difficult to understand where Frey and Singer differ in method, even though they differ radically in their conclusions. Frey believes that animal research must pass a test similar to the one described by Singer. Frey believes that it would be wrong to perform an experiment on an animal if we were not willing to perform it on a human with an even lower potential quality of life (e.g., an orphaned infant born without a brain). However, Frey recognizes the benefits which flow from animal research and seems intent on preserving them. Therefore, while he maintains that we should be willing to perform such human experiments, he also recognizes reasons why we might choose not to. The "side effects" of such human research (like societal uproar, outraged relatives, etc.) may outweigh the benefits derived, and thereby cause us to refrain from conducting them in the first place.

Singer's claim that speciesism is analogous to racism has also received criticism. Peter Carruthers, a British philosopher and supporter of animal research, believes that species membership is a morally relevant characteristic (9), as do Stephen Post of Case Western Reserve University (38) and Carl Cohen of the University of Michigan (10). Animal rights philosopher Mary Midgley, who is clearly willing to demand limitations on the use of animals in research (32,33), also rejects the speciesism–racism analogy. She argues that "race in humans is not a significant grouping at all, but species in animals certainly is. It is never true that, in order to know how to treat a human being, you must first find out what race he belongs to.... But with an animal, to know the species is absolutely essential" (35). For Midgley there are morally significant bonds which exist between species members just as between the members of a family. However, these species bonds are not absolute, and it is important to realize that we also form significant bonds with members of other species (34).

Deontology

The second of the two major categories of ethical thought, deontology, does not depend exclusively on the consequences of an action to determine its morality. This does not necessarily mean that consequences play no role whatsoever in deontological theories. Those theories which admit to the relevance of consequences, in addition to other considerations, have been referred to as "moderate" theories, while theories which maintain that consequences must not be considered at all are called "extreme." The best-known deontological theory is that developed by the German philosopher Immanuel Kant (1724–1804). His theory is an example of an extreme deontological position in that the consequences of an action are not considered in establishing its morality. Kant believed that using the utility of an act to determine whether it was right or wrong was a terrible mistake. He realized, as we have already seen, that such a standard compels the moral person to perform a particular act in one situation, while forbidding it in another. This changing standard of morality was unacceptable to Kant, and so he developed a theory based on a principle which, unlike utility, would not change from one situation to another.

The principle which Kant developed to accomplish this purpose is called the Categorical Imperative. Kant formulated this principle in a number of different ways which he maintained were all equivalent

(31). One of these advises us to "act only on that maxim through which you can at the same time will that it should become a universal law." How does this principle guide and constrain our actions? In order to determine if a particular act is moral, we must first ask ourselves if we could wish that the rule governing our action be made a universal law—that is, if we would wish for everybody to follow the same course of action. If we cannot truthfully desire that anyone else be permitted to perform the action that we are considering, that act is immoral.

Let's, once again, suppose that you are considering lying about the results of certain experiments that you have performed. Before doing this, the Categorical Imperative requires that you first ask yourself whether or not you can honestly wish that your deed be universalized into a rule. This rule would permit all scientists to submit fraudulent data as genuine. Clearly such a rule would destroy the credibility of all scientists, and preclude the ability of the scientific community to make organized advances (as well as having much broader implications for the general concept of truthfulness). No one could legitimately wish that such a rule be universalized—therefore the act is immoral. Note that there was no consideration of the consequences of your contemplated act of deception. Whether or not you might benefit from your deed never entered into the moral calculus.

A second formulation of Kant's Categorical Imperative is more frequently encountered in discussions of medical ethics (31). This formulation advises us to "act in such a way that you always treat humanity, whether in your own person or in the person of any other, never simply as a means, but always at the same time as an end." This statement makes it more clear that Kant's principle also requires a certain respect for persons. Notice that Kant does not demand that we *never* use a person as a means to an end, just that we do not use a person *solely* as a means. When a physician treats paying patients, she is clearly using them as a means through which she can achieve an end for herself (earning a living). Yet if this is the physician's sole consideration in treating patients, she will be acting immorally toward them. Patients, and all other persons, are to be treated as ends as well as means. Patients have interests independent of those of the physician from whom they have sought treatment. In other words, patients are their own ends. A physician who prescribes "snake oil" is acting immorally because she fails to treat the patient as an end. The physician who provides her patients with the best care available treats them as both a means and an end.

Regan's deontology and animal rights

Tom Regan is a professor of philosophy at North Carolina State University and the author of *The Case for Animal Rights* (39). Whereas Singer rejects the philosophical concept of "rights," Regan embraces it. He describes "the rights view" as a type of deontological theory distinct from that articulated by Kant.

> According to this theory, certain individuals have moral rights (e.g., the right to life) and they have these rights independently of considerations about the value of the consequences that would flow from recognizing that they have them. For the rights view in other words, rights are more basic than utility and independent of it, so that the principle reason why, say, murder is wrong, if and when it is, lies in the violation of the victim's moral right to life, and not in considerations about who will or will not receive pleasure or pain or have their preferences satisfied or frustrated, as a result of the deed. Those who subscribe to the rights view need not hold that all moral rights are absolute in the sense that they can never be overridden by other moral considerations. For example, one could hold that when the only realistic way to respect the rights of the many is to override the moral rights of the few, then overriding these rights is justified. (39)

In his rejection of utilitarian ethics, Regan charges that consequentialist philosophies make a mistake in viewing individuals as little more than a receptacle to be filled with pleasure or displeasure. Regan's analogy is that of a cup filled with either a sweet liquid, a bitter liquid, or some combination of the two. He maintains that utilitarians ignore the value of the cup (the individual) and only concentrate on the liquid within it (pleasure or displeasure). Regan argues that individuals themselves possess a property which he calls "inherent value." Inherent value, according to Regan, is not dependent on the race, sex, religion, or birthplace of an individual. Further, it does not depend on the intelligence, talents, skills, or importance of a person. "The genius and the retarded child, the prince and the pauper, the brain surgeon and the fruit vendor, Mother Teresa and the most unscrupulous used car salesman—all have inherent value, all possess it equally, and all have an equal right to be treated with respect, to be treated in ways that do not reduce them to the status of things, as if they existed as resources for others" (40). Regan also claims that it would be blatant speciesism to insist that only humans have inherent value. He argues that many animals also possess it. But how does he decide which animals possess inherent value and which animals do not? Regan's test for the possession of inherent value is something he terms the "subject of a life criterion." This does not require that one merely be alive but that also that one "have beliefs and desires; perception, memory, and a sense of the future, including their own future, an emotional life together with feeling of pleasure and pain; preference- and welfare-interests; the ability to initiate action in pursuit of their desires and goals; a psychophysical identity over time; and an individual welfare in the sense that their experiential life fares well or ill for them...." (39). At the time he wrote *The Case for Animal Rights* Regan seemed to think that all mammals over the age of one year possess inherent value. In more recent statements, he seems to believe that this range should be expanded considerably.

The claim that animals have inherent value seems to agree with our sense of moral intuition and up to this point many of you may have found little to argue with. However, Regan's insistence that inherent value is a "categorical concept" is likely to prove more controversial. What Regan means by this is that humans cannot be said to possess any more inherent value than any other animal. Either animals are in the category of beings that possess inherent value or they are not. "One either has it, or one does not. There are no in-betweens. Moreover, all those who have it, have it equally. It does not come in degrees" (39). When pressed to delineate the exact point of demarcation between those beings said to possess inherent value and those that do not, Regan deflects the question as essentially moot. "Whether it belongs to others—to rocks and rivers, trees and glaciers, for example—we do not know and may never know. But neither do we need to know, if we are to make the case for animal rights. We do not need to know, for example, how many people are eligible to vote in the next presidential election before we can know whether I am" (40). But Regan's position does not imply that he believes that there are no moral differences between animals and humans. If there are five individuals (four humans and a dog) who seek sanctuary in a lifeboat which can hold only four of them what should be done? Regan believes that it is the dog who should be thrown overboard to die. He argues that while the inherent value of each of these beings is equivalent, the harm which would be done to them through their deaths is not. Humans have a much greater range of possibilities open to them in their lives than do dogs. Humans can experience joys and satisfactions which no dog will ever experience. Because of this, death forecloses far more potential opportunities for satisfaction in the human than it will in the dog. Regan argues that it would be allowable to throw even one million dogs overboard to save the humans because each dog's death, when considered one at a time, is less harmful than the death of a human considered one at a time.

One might imagine, from such a position, that Regan would be disposed to permit animal research which could save the lives of humans. However, Regan's position is, if anything, more severe than is Singer's on the question of animal research. Regan states that his ethic requires the immediate abolition of all such research. Why isn't medical research seen as analogous to the lifeboat ethics described above? In the lifeboat example, all (including the dog) would have perished if one individual was not sacrificed. A decision had to be made as to whether it was a human or a dog that had to die so that the others could live. Regan does not see that choice as analogous to using animals in research on human disease. The animals are not in the lifeboat because they are not sick. No decision has to be made to sacrifice one or the other. In Kantian terms one can imagine that Regan believes that medical research uses animals merely as a means and not also as an end.

While Regan is quite comfortable with his abolitionist position, it should be noted that he, like Singer, does not seem to view the loss of the ability to use animals in research as having grave consequences for medical advances. Regan writes, "Like Galileo's contemporaries, who would not look through the telescope because they had already convinced themselves of what they would see and thus saw no need to look, those scientists who have convinced themselves that there can't be viable scientific alternatives to the use of whole animals in research (or toxicity tests, etc.) are captives of mental habits that true science abhors" (39).

Regan's views have also been extensively criticized. The utilitarian philosopher and cautious supporter of animal research R. G. Frey questions the claim that animals have moral rights. As a utilitarian Frey doubts the existence of moral rights in the first place, but his criticism extends beyond his philosophical viewpoint. (It can be hypothesized that Frey's criticism of the philosophical concept of rights would be largely echoed by Peter Singer.) Frey notes that the concept of moral rights is especially popular in the United States and that, in this country, the position in contentious social issues is often stated in rights language (women's rights, gay rights, children's rights). Often the opposing sides in a debate will each make appeals using rights language—the "right to life" versus "a woman's right to choose." Frey argues that, in the United States, for a group "to fail to cast its wants in terms of rights...is to disadvantage itself in this debate..." (20). In contrast, he observes that debates over the moral treatment of animals have proceeded in Britain and Australia with relatively little mention of rights.

Carl Cohen has argued that animals are not the kind of creatures capable of possessing rights (10). He states that rights can only be accorded to "beings who actually do, or can, make moral claims against one another." Carruthers criticizes Regan on a much more fundamental level (9). He claims that Regan has not adequately provided a groundwork for his moral theory. Where are the rights he argues for supposed to have come from? What exactly is the "inherent value" which Regan claims is possessed (at least) by all mammals of one year of age or older? How do we detect inherent value; that is, how are we to determine which life forms have it and which do not? Carruthers accuses Regan of altogether failing to provide the kind of "governing conception" necessary to explain his moral theory.

Practical Matters: Constraints on the Behavior of Scientists

We have seen that there is no unanimity among those philosophers critical of the use of animals in biomedical research. Likewise, there is no unanimity among the philosophers who support such use. R. G. Frey (19–22), Peter Carruthers (9), Michael P. T. Leahy (29), and Carl Cohen (10) each argues from his own philosophical perspective. So while these readings can provide us with useful frameworks for thinking about ethical problems, those hoping for a simple consensus view on why it is morally permissible to experiment on animals will be just as disappointed as those hoping for a consensus supporting the opposite view. But we do not require a confluence of philosophical opinion to recognize that the use of animals in research entails a moral responsibility.

Legislation

Scientists no longer have the luxury, or burden, of being the sole arbiter of the acceptability of their own experiments. In the early days of animal research, scientists had little to restrict their use of animals other than their own individual consciences. This is not the case today. Discuss animal care with any of the older scientists, or with animal care technicians with whom you work, and they will tell you how dramatically the definition of what constitutes "acceptable" treatment has changed over the years. Scientists work under a number of restrictions—legal, institutional, and moral—which constrain how animals may be used in experiments.

In 1963, the National Institutes of Health (NIH) published its first *Guide for the Care and Use of Laboratory Animals*. At first, compliance with the recommendations set out in the guide was voluntary. The movement to pass restrictive legislation gained momentum in early 1966 when an article in *Life* magazine (1) caused public outrage by chronicling the despicable conditions under which many animal dealers maintained their dogs (36,41). In August of 1966, Congress passed the Laboratory Animal Welfare Act. A major goal of this legislation was to require the registration of research facilities, and dog dealers, with the U.S. Department of Agriculture (USDA). A clear intent of the bill was to minimize the number of instances where people's cats and dogs were stolen and sold to research institutions. These institutions were now required to buy their cats and dogs from licensed dealers. This legislation was amended in 1970, 1976, and 1985, and is now referred to as the Animal Welfare Act. The legislation mandated humane care and treatment for dogs, cats, rabbits, hamsters, guinea pigs, and nonhuman primates. However, it provided no protection for rats and mice, the two species which account for the vast majority of all animals used in research.

Shortly before the last set of amendments to the Animal Welfare Act was instituted, Congress passed the Health Research Extension Act of 1985 (Public Law 99-158). This was the first law concerning animals under which the U.S. Public Health Service (USPHS) was required to operate. This law, in effect, caused the heretofore voluntary

Public Health Service Policy on the Humane Care and Use of Laboratory Animals (3) to become mandatory for both USPHS research labs and any nongovernmental institutions that received funding from any USPHS agency. The USPHS policy includes a number of key elements, one of which is an assurance obtained from research institutions stating that they are committed to following the USPHS policy and the *Guide for the Care and Use of Laboratory Animals* (2).

The *Guide for the Care and Use of Laboratory Animals,* often referred to simply as "the *Guide,*" is an important document for scientists and animal care personnel. The *Guide* describes details on how animal research should be carried out within an institution. Although the Animal Welfare Act does not itself address rats and mice, the *Guide* does include these species. It details a number of institutional policies which should be put into place concerning issues such as the qualifications and training of the professional animal care staff and the establishment of an occupational health program to protect personnel who come into contact with the animals. Other special considerations include policies discouraging the prolonged physical restraint of animals and the use of multiple major surgical procedures on a single animal. The *Guide* also addresses issues surrounding the animal facilities and housing requirements for experimental animals. Minimum space recommendations are given in detail for a number of different species. (For example, it is suggested that a 20-gram mouse be allotted at least 12 square inches of floor space in a cage that is at least 5 inches high.) Further, it is recommended that attention be given to the particular social requirements of the animal species in question. Communal animals should be housed in groups whenever appropriate, while taking into account things such as population density, familiarity of individuals, and social rank. For highly social animals (such as dogs and nonhuman primates), it is suggested that group composition be held as stable as possible. It is also suggested that the environment of the animals be enriched to prevent boredom, especially when animals are to be held for a long period of time.

The physical environment under which the animals are maintained is also addressed in the *Guide.* Temperature and humidity ranges are given for a number of species, as well as suggestions for ventilating animals' rooms (10 to 15 room air changes per hour). Levels of illumination are suggested because light which is within the comfortable range for humans can actually be so bright that it damages the retinas of albino mice. In addition, the *Guide* discusses noise levels and requirements for bedding, water, sanitation, waste disposal, and vermin control. Veterinary care issues such as quarantine, separation by species, and disease control are discussed, as are anesthesia, surgical and postsurgical care, and recommended means of euthanasia. The *Guide* also addresses many aspects of the actual physical plant in which animals are housed and experimented upon. Recommendations are given for corridor sizes, animal room door sizes, ceiling heights, placement of floor drains, the surface material from which the walls should be constructed, and suggested locations of storage areas for food and bedding.

Additionally, the USPHS policy requires the establishment of Institutional Animal Care and Use Committees (IACUCs) which oversee the animal care and use program (ACU) for the institution. The IACUC comprises at least five members, including a veterinarian with experience or training in laboratory animal medicine, a practicing scientist experienced in animal research, a nonscientist, and an individual who is not affiliated with the institution in any way other than as a member of the IACUC. Typically IACUCs are larger than the minimum size required and may have 10 or more members. The IACUC is charged with evaluating the ACU and animal facilities every six months and preparing a report on its findings. It also evaluates and makes recommendations regarding all aspects of an institution's animal research program, including training of personnel. The IACUC has the authority to suspend any activity at an institution which involves animals should it determine that the research is not being conducted in accordance with the Animal Welfare Act or the *Guide for the Care and Use of Laboratory Animals*.

Another extremely important role of the IACUC is the review of animal welfare concerns of research protocols submitted by individual institutional scientists. The submitted protocol describes the species of animal proposed to be used, the details of the experimental procedures, the types of anesthesia or analgesia which will be used for painful procedures, and what method of euthanasia will be used to terminate the experiment. The IACUC considers the qualifications and training of the principal investigators and their staff members in addition to the details of the protocol when making its decision. IACUC approval of the research protocol is required before an NIH grant can be funded and is to be obtained before *any* experiments are started.

When reviewing an investigator's research protocol, the IACUC must determine whether the proposed experiments are being conducted in accordance with the Animal Welfare Act and the *Guide for the Care and Use of Laboratory Animals*. Any departures from these guidelines must be justified by the scientist to the satisfaction of the committee. The committee is to ensure that protocols are designed to avoid or minimize discomfort, distress, and pain to animals consistent with sound research design. Any procedure which is judged to cause more than a "momentary or slight pain or distress" should be performed with appropriate sedation, analgesia, or anesthesia unless the investigator can convince the committee that withholding such treatment is justified for scientific reasons. Animals that would suffer severe or chronic pain and distress which cannot be relieved must be euthanized. The committee must also ensure that the experimental animals covered by a particular protocol will be housed under conditions which are appropriate for the species and which will contribute to "their health and comfort" (3). The housing, feeding, and nonmedical care of the animals must be directed by a veterinarian or other scientist trained and experienced in the care of the species being used. Medical care for the animals must be provided by a qualified veterinarian. Any means of euthanasia employed must be consistent with the recommendations of the American Veterinary Medical Association Panel on Euthanasia unless the investigator is able to justify any deviation on scientific grounds to the satisfaction of the IACUC. In recent years, there has been increasing thought given to how one might assign ethical scores to animal protocols (36,37). While this may be difficult to do with great precision, it is clear that the committee can usually agree on those proposals which are the most problematic with relative ease. The IACUC is not restricted to simply accepting or rejecting the investigator's protocol. Often the IACUC will suggest alterations to a protocol which would make it acceptable. The committee may suggest a different anesthetic, or perhaps an alternative dose or schedule of treatment. The IACUC can draw upon the expertise of its various members in order to work with the investigator to see that both scientific and animal welfare concerns are met. Occasionally investigators feel that the suggestions of the IACUC are intrusions into their scientific experimental design. This is unfortunate, but it is nonetheless the responsibility of the committee to ensure that all animal welfare concerns are satisfied. An investigator's attempt to justify a particular technique by using the argument that "this is the way that we have always done it" is not a sufficient rationale for an IACUC to approve a protocol which might otherwise be questionable. Likewise, it is also not a sufficient rationale to claim that similar (or identical) techniques have been approved for use at other institutions. Each IACUC is responsible for making decisions on the protocols which come before it and differences of opinion from one institution to another as to the acceptability of a particular technique are bound to occur.

Another important element of the USPHS policy is the requirement that the institution provide training for those staff members involved in the care and / or research use of animals. This training is to include a discussion of humane methods of animal care and experimentation, techniques available to minimize the use of animals and animal distress, the proper use of anesthetics and analgesics, methods by which deficient animal care procedures might be reported, and how to use available services to learn more about appropriate animal care and alternatives to animal techniques. The National Research Council has prepared a book to assist in the development of such institutional programs (4).

Although the Animal Welfare Act has not been legislatively amended since 1985, some have attempted to alter the scope and specifics of the act through judicial action. Since the inception of the Animal Welfare Act in 1966, the USDA has excluded rats, mice, and birds from being covered under its regulations. After failing to persuade the USDA to amend these regulations, the Animal Legal Defense Fund (ALDF) brought suit in 1990 to force the inclusion of rats, mice, and birds. In January 1992, U.S. District Court Judge Charles Richey ruled in favor of the ALDF. In his decision, Judge Richey wrote that the USDA "violated the mandate of the Federal Laboratory Animal Welfare Act...by promulgating regulations which fail to include birds, rats, and mice as 'animals' within the meaning of the act" (50). Judge Richey also charged that the "agency's interpretation of the statute is arbitrary and capricious."

A little more that one year later, Judge Richey once again issued an opinion on the Animal Welfare Act in response to a lawsuit brought by the ALDF and Society for Protective Animal Legislation (51). In this opinion, he ruled that the USDA had failed to implement the 1985 amendments to the Animal Welfare Act. These amendments included provisions that stated that dogs were to receive opportunities for exercise and that measures were to be taken to improve the psychological well-being of primates. The USDA wrote what are known as "performance-based standards" when it instructed research facilities to implement these requirements in accordance with "currently accepted professional standards." The judge ruled that this instruction amounted to allowing the research facilities to police themselves and hence violated the law. The judge ordered the USDA to implement a set of "minimum requirements" with which all research facilities must comply. What the animal welfare groups desire, and the judge is ordering, is a set of what are referred to as "engineering standards." These would involve very specific minimum requirements for compliance with the law. An earlier version of the USDA's instructions had mandated that dogs be walked for 30 minutes per day. In the final version, research institutions were instructed to allow the dogs "the opportunity" for "regular exercise." Judge Richey wrote that such an instruction was in essence allowing minimum level of care to depend on "good faith compliance by the regulated entities" (8).

In May and July of 1994, the U.S. Court of Appeals for the District of Columbia overturned Judge Richey's two decisions. The Appeals Court ruled that the parties which brought the suit did not have legal standing to do so and, because of this, Judge Richey's federal court had no jurisdiction to make a ruling. While this particular attempt to alter the Animal Welfare Act through judicial action appears to have failed, it is important not to think of the act as a static document. The Animal Welfare Act has been amended in the past and it is certain to be modified again in the future, whether by legislation or by lawsuit.

Given the current legal climate, it may be impossible for any book to present an up-to-date assessment of the laws regulating the care and use of laboratory animals. For current information, scientists will have to depend on the Division of Animal Resources within their own research institutions. As we will discuss below, the relationship between animal care professionals and scientists is going to become increasingly important.

Beyond legislation
While laws define the minimum required of scientists in the care and use of animals, most scientists will want to strive for levels of care which exceed these minimums. The scientist's primary ally in this goal

is the institution's Division of Animal Care or equivalent body. The veterinarians and animal care professionals employed by this department serve as a powerful resource to scientists. Using their knowledge can lead to both better animal care and better science.

In most instances, it will be these professionals who provide the training which is now mandated by law for those who are going to use animals in their research. New graduate students should be sure that they attend these training sessions as early as possible. Traditionally, the training in animal procedures for new graduate students has taken place within the laboratory of their chosen advisor. However, animal care professionals are better able to provide a comprehensive training experience than the old *ad hoc* system in place in most laboratories. In addition to this formal training experience, students should realize that their institution's animal care professionals can also be an invaluable resource when they are seeking to learn a new procedure or technique. In addition to being able to advise you as to what is required by law when, for example, performing rodent surgery, they will also be able to advise you on the appropriate surgical techniques, use of anesthetics, and postoperative care. This advice can ensure both that the experimental animal does not suffer any unnecessary pain or distress and that you obtain the best data possible from your experimental efforts.

Although it is the legal responsibility of the faculty advisor (principal investigator) to submit protocols to the IACUC, students would be well advised to look at the protocols under which they are conducting their research. Laboratory techniques often drift over time as personnel and experience change. Graduate students are likely in a better position than are their advisors to see this happening and realize that it is time to submit an amended protocol to the IACUC. Additionally, scientists are required to consider the use of nonanimal alternative techniques before resorting to the use of animals for any procedure likely to cause pain or distress. Senior graduate and postdoctoral students are often on the cutting edge of technology and thus in an excellent position to make suggestions to their advisor for improving laboratory procedures. In 1959, Russell and Burch suggested three principles which they suggested act as a guide for the humane use of animals in research (42). These are commonly referred to as the three R's: "Replacement, Reduction, and Refinement."

- *Replacement* refers to the attempt to substitute insentient materials, or if this is not possible, a lower species which might be less susceptible to pain and distress than a higher species. Why sacrifice the life a monkey for an experiment in which a dog would suffice? Why use a dog where a mouse would do? Why use a mouse if the research question could be answered using a cell culture?
- *Reduction* refers to the attempt to use the minimum number of animal lives necessary to answer the research question. To design an experiment in which the n of a treatment group is 25 in a situation where statistical significance could be achieved with an $n = 8$ is both economically wasteful and morally troubling. However, it is equally troubling to see an experimental design where too few animals are used. If the group size were too small to permit any reasonable chance of demonstrating a statistically significant difference, then the entire experiment would be a wasted effort. There are techniques available to assist in the estimation of the appropriate numbers of animals to be used in an experiment (30). Additionally, one can seek the advice of a professional statistician prior to conducting a series of experiments both to prevent the wasting of animal lives and to ensure a more rigorous scientific study.
- *Refinement* refers to the attempt to reduce the incidence or severity of pain and distress experienced by experimental animals. Use of anesthetics and analgesics which are appropriate for the experimental species, as well as the use of the appropriate doses and intervals of administration, are all important. Additionally, use of trained personnel to perform experimental or surgical manipulations and effective postoperative procedures will improve both animal welfare and scientific validity. (Who would want pain introduced as an uncontrolled variable into their experimental design?)

Finally it should be recognized that animal care professionals play something of a dual role within the institution. As we have discussed, they can serve as an invaluable resource to the research scientist. However they also must ensure the welfare of the animals under their care. This role could potentially put them at odds with the research scientist. The animal care staff is also there to protect the animals from any researcher who refuses to observe the rules. This dual role can be stressful, as they are at the same time advocates for both scientific research and animal welfare. For a more detailed examination of the ambivalent feelings experienced by some animal care personnel and scientific staff, a series of articles written by sociologist Arnold Arluke is recommended (5–7).

We should recognize that while the work we do is important and morally justified in the minds of most people, our system is not perfect and there are ways in which we can contribute to improved animal care. Each of us should be on the lookout for animals who are suffering, either from neglect or from abuse at the hands of a careless or poorly trained scientist. In some instances, the situation might be resolved by talking to the person involved. In other situations, a report might have to be made (formally or anonymously) to the head veterinarian of the animal care staff.

In addition it is also beneficial for us to realize that there are moral inconsistencies in the way scientists relate to animals. Harold Herzog has written provocatively on this matter. He wonders why it is that we have strict rules for how we may use and euthanize laboratory mice, and yet be allowed to catch and kill escaped mice in in humane "sticky traps" (25). After once being accused (unjustly) by an animal activist of obtaining kittens from a local animal pound in order to feed his son's boa constrictor, Herzog began to think about the ethics of pet food (27). Is it more moral to raise a rat to feed to a boa than it is to use a kitten which is about to die anyway? For that matter, is it any more moral to keep a kitten (an obligate carnivore) than it is a boa? Herzog's articles provide an intriguing stimulus to thinking about the animals we choose to keep in our homes as well as those we use in research (23,24,26).

Political Realities: Then and Now

The political realities are such that there is no chance that scientists will be left to decide by themselves how laboratory animal welfare may be improved. The last 15 years has seen the rise of a number of well-funded animal rights groups that can be expected to press for legislative and judicial mandates to alter the existing procedures. While some of these initiatives will originate from a genuine concern to improve the treatment of laboratory animals, others seek to harass animal research until such a time that the groups believe that they will amass the political might to see such research abolished. While scientists often like to believe that the animals rights movement consists of a lunatic fringe, such an assertion is not true and carries with it a great danger. (For who seriously worries about the demented rambling of a group of lunatics?) Apart from a few apparently irrational statements made by the leaders of some animal rights groups, there is no evidence that the membership is anything other than a group of highly concerned citizens. It is important that we set aside the easy (and erroneous) explanations of the animal rights phenomenon and seriously consider who is involved in the movement and why.

The "first" public antivivisectionist movement was initiated in Victorian England by well-connected, politically sophisticated, affluent people during the middle of the 19th century. They had access to the highest levels of the government, including the sympathies of Queen Victoria, and were capable of mounting effective public relations campaigns. The same is certainly true of the new "animals rights" movement today. A recent survey of animal rights activists attending a march in Washington, D.C. revealed a level of political activity which was termed "truly extraordinary" (28). The fact that 74% of those surveyed had contacted their elected representatives about animal rights, and that 38% had made political donations to candidates supportive of such rights, suggests a highly motivated and politically sophisticated activist group. The fact that nearly 14% of the activists reported having incomes in excess of $70,000 per year, and more than 30% in excess of $50,000 per year, helps to explain why the animal rights movement is so well funded. Like the Victorian antivivisectionists who preceded them, the modern animal rights activists are well educated—nearly 79% reported some college education, 47% a bachelor's degree, and nearly 19% a graduate or professional degree.

The Victorian antivivisection movement represented a significant break with the existing humane movement of that time. The traditional humane organizations were essentially conservative groups dedicated to reform through education and legislation. These groups were supportive of social norms, despite their demands for improved treatment of animals. However, the antivivisectionist groups pressed for changes on a more fundamental level, changes which required modification of existing social norms (48). The same distinction can be made today between those groups which are concerned primarily with the humane treatment of animals and those which press for radical alterations in the predominant world view. Not surprisingly, these more radical beliefs sometimes lead to internal inconsistencies between the leaders of the movement and the rank-and-file membership over issues such as the morality of pet ownership (28).

The Victorian movement was plagued by internal strife and struggle. Historian Richard French writes, "From the institutional origins of the movement to the twentieth century, then, the atmosphere within it was soured by disharmony and disunity. Differences between various societies, publications, and individual workers were ostensibly rooted in questions of policy and tactics. But jealousy, personal ambition, and especially the desire for public attention in a leadership role, were at least as important as more substantive issues in motivating the disputes that fragmented organized antivivisection—and any number of other reforming agitations. Discussion of ends and means could never be effectively disentangled from the clash of personality and ego. What was at stake was as much career as conviction" (18). Likewise, the modern animal rights movement has been plagued by internal squabbling over issues ranging from differences in fundamental philosophy to those of excessive executive salaries.

Many of the Victorian activists were ambivalent about science and the role it was assuming in society. Science was viewed by some as an assault on religious faith, morality, and nature (13,49). The new scientific medicine with its emphasis on the physical basis of disease challenged the link between morality and good health. For some antivivisectionists, disease was seen as the result of sin and moral turpitude. The fact that many prostitutes had venereal disease was thought to be just, and to intervene in these cases was interference with divine retribution (49). Likewise, the use of anesthetics during childbirth was feared by some to be an unjustified obstruction of the divine punishment inflicted on women because of "original sin" (17,47). While such views seem incredible to those of us with a modern biological understanding of disease, they nevertheless help to explain a portion of the horror with which many antivivisectionists viewed modern medicine and the discoveries which are today judged as beneficial.

Although they are not usually expressed in religious terms, the modern animal rights movement also displays profound doubts about scientific enterprise. Fifty-two percent of animal rights activists surveyed felt that science does "more harm than good." This opinion sets them dramatically apart from the general public wherein only 5% expresses this belief. The activists view scientists in the same suspicious light reserved for other traditional authority figures such as politicians and businessmen (28).

Further, it is a mistake to believe that this skepticism is limited to the benefits derived from scientific research or to the character of the scientists performing such work. Gary Francione, professor of law at Rutgers University and former legal advisor to People for the Ethical Treatment of Animals (PETA), has expressed mistrust of the scientific process itself.

> ...science no longer enjoys a position as epistemologically superior to other forms of knowledge. Despite the seductive simplicity of the traditional empiricist point of view—that science represents "objective" truth—the assumptions supporting this traditional view have been challenged effectively in recent years. Philosophers and sociologists of science have argued persuasively that factual assertions are completely contingent on theoretical assumptions, and that observation itself is subject to interpretation....
>
> This recognition is slowly eroding the pedestal upon which science has presided for many years. More and more people in the animal rights movement, the environmental movement, and the alternative health care movement recognize that science is as value-based as any other activity. Indeed, there is increasing criticism of the fundamental premises of Western medicine. (16)

Francione has also written to challenge the "general view" that scientific inquiry is protected under the First Amendment to the United States Constitution. Francione's view is that the First Amendment provides very little protection to the conduct of scientific research although, somewhat paradoxically, the dissemination of the research results themselves is protected. "For example, under this analysis, the government could...prohibit all research involving genetic engineering as long as the purpose of the prohibition is not to suppress the dissemination of the information derived from such research" (14).

While it is not clear that Professor Francione would be in favor of prohibiting all genetic engineering research, there is little doubt that he opposes all use of animals in scientific research. In another law review article, Francione criticizes the regulatory reforms proposed by law professor Rebecca Dresser. Professor Dresser suggests that scientists be required to perform a more rigorous risk/benefit analysis, as is mandated in the human research approval process, before receiving approval to use animals in their research (11). Francione objects because Dresser seems to accept that "there are convincing legal reasons for postulating" First Amendment protections to the right to conduct animal research. Statements made in Professor Francione's concluding paragraph give us some insight as to why he appears to be so opposed to the concept of Constitutional protections for research.

> It may be the case, however, that the federal government will, at some point, try to impose on all experimentation a risk/benefit regulatory structure similar to the one that Professor Dresser proposes. *Moreover, it is likely that even though experimenters find themselves with the federal (or other) funds to do an experiment, state and local governments may seek to restrict or even to prohibit such experimentation....* (15) (emphasis added)

We may be seeing in such statements a strategy for political action from a movement which has been unable to convince a majority of society as to the legitimacy of its views. While over the past 18 years the animal rights movement has succeeded in causing increasing numbers of the public to question both the validity and humanity of animal research, it has at the same time failed to build anything approaching a consensus for animal "rights" as it conceives of them. Thus it seems possible that in the future the movement may try to achieve, through targeted political actions in state and local arenas, what it has been unable to win through philosophical debate at the national level. Given the political savvy of the movement, this would not appear to be an idle threat. (Francione himself clerked for Supreme Court Justice Sandra Day O'Connor after completing law school.) While there is no hope, in the foreseeable future, of the movement securing a legal prohibition of animal research at the national level, things seem less certain at the level of local government. Imagine the impact of a local ordinance proscribing animal research within the city limits of a community such as Berkeley, California, or Cambridge, Massachusetts. The ordinance may not even be phrased in the philosophical terms of animal rights, but rather may appear to be primarily concerned with the alleged environmental impact, or health risks to citizens, associated with animal research.

Given the political, financial, and human resources available to the animal rights movement, it seems unlikely that socially responsible scientists will be able to conform to our society's stereotypical view of scientists—cloistered away in our labs, working night and day, oblivious to the political realities of the world around us. The extent to which any scientist decides to become involved in the political and philosophical debate over animal rights is a matter of individual choice. Nevertheless, all scientists have an obligation to educate themselves about this issue, both to ensure ever-increasing standards of animal welfare as well as to ensure that society will continue to seek their counsel when searching for answers to this ethical dilemma.

Case Studies

5.1 A graduate student asks a faculty member if he or she would like to observe something "interesting." When the faculty member assents, the student quickly injects a mouse with a large volume (10+ ml) of air and puts the bloated, twitching mouse on the lab bench to observe. You are the faculty member, and upon investigation, learn that the graduate student has performed this "demonstration" for a number of other students and technicians. What do you do?

5.2 A graduate faculty advisor has a predoctoral trainee in his laboratory who needs to raise antibodies in rabbits in order to analyze a specific protein. No one in the laboratory has ever used animals or antibodies in their research. The advisor instructs the student to do the necessary "homework" and determine what is needed to prepare a proposed protocol for approval by the institutional animal use committee. The predoctoral trainee does as directed and prepares and types the entire application herself. The predoctoral trainee presents the completed document to her advisor who, in turn, reads and signs the document. He hands it back to the student instructing her to submit it to the animal care committee office for review. The mentor commends the student for the work and comments that this has been an important "learning experience" for the student. Comment on the mentor's responsibilities and actions in this matter.

5.3 You are a graduate student working on your Ph.D. Your advisor asks to meet with you to discuss your research project. Your advisor suggests a new series of experiments which will hopefully clear up a problem you have encountered. The new series of experiments involves surgical manipulations and, having read the IACUC protocol for the project, you know that it did not contain any reference to surgery. You ask your advisor about submitting an amended protocol before starting these studies. Your advisor says that he does not wish to go through the trouble if the technique is not going to be useful. He suggests that you first try a few experiments and, if the procedure looks like it is going to work and you will continue performing it, you can submit an amended protocol at that time. What do you do?

5.4 A faculty member is conducting institutionally approved, NIH-sponsored animal research that involves a surgical technique performed on adult rats. Control rats from such experiments are mildly sedated during the procedure but receive no other medicinal treatment. They are sacrificed at the end of the experiment and again examined with a minor surgical technique. An owner of a pet store approaches the faculty member and asks if he can have the sacrificed control rats to use as food for his boa constrictor snakes. The pet store owner suggests that the faculty member file an addendum to his animal use authorization form to seek permission to give him the rat carcasses. The faculty member comes to you for advice. What advice do you give him?

5.5 A colleague of yours is going to appear at a career day held at a local school. She will use mice to illustrate the effects of various psychoactive drugs (including drugs of abuse) to the children. The mice will be used in various experiments for which she has IACUC approval to perform in her lab. The experiments involve such endpoints as loss of balance, flicking of the tail out of the path of an uncomfortably warm light beam, and other standard assays. She wonders whether or not she should seek IACUC approval for this special appearance at the career day. She is worried that the IACUC approval may not come in time, and the submission represents a considerable amount of work. What would you advise?

5.6 You are a member of an NIH study section and you are in the process of reviewing grants for an upcoming meeting. One of your primary assignments involves a grant where rabbits will be used to raise antibodies. In reading over the protocol, you discover that the investigator will perform repeated bleedings of these animals to recover enough antiserum to do his experiments. The rabbits will not be sacrificed and exsanguinated to recover the maximum amount of blood at the end of the experiment. Instead, the investigator states that the rabbits will be given away as pets at the end of the experiment. Is this proposal appropriate? If you are troubled by this proposal, what would you proceed to do?

5.7 You are invited as a guest faculty member to judge a local high school science fair. One entry you judge is entitled "Alcohol Addiction in Mice." The student has purchased six mice from a local pet store. One group of three of these mice has been caged and fed standard mouse chow and given drinking water ad libitum. The other group is fed mouse chow but is allowed water only once per day. This group of mice is instead given unlimited access to 20% ethyl alcohol. After six weeks, the student notes a significant weight loss in the latter group of mice as compared with the control animals. He also notes abdominal distension and states that the alcohol-fed mice ate significantly less food throughout the study. He concludes that the alcohol mixture depressed the animals' appetites. At the end of the study, he destroys the animals by cervical dislocation. You consult the school guidelines regarding the use of animals in science projects. The guidelines state that animal use in science projects is discouraged. However, animals may be used with permission of the science teacher. In this case, the student has sought and received such permission for his project. What comments, if any, will you offer to the student about his use of animals? Likewise, what, it anything, will you say to his teacher?

5.8 You are a member of your institution's IACUC. A protocol is submitted in which a researcher plans to perform some surgical manipulations on mice under anesthesia and then allow them to recover. The investigator does not wish to use any analgesics on the mice after they regain consciousness for fear that the drugs will alter the immune responses she is seeking to measure. No data are provided to show that analgesic drugs alter immunity. Would you vote to approve this protocol? If not, what would your advice to the investigator be?

5.9 You are a member of your institution's IACUC. A protocol is submitted in which a researcher plans to perform footpad injections in mice using an antigen in complete Freund's adjuvant (CFA) in order to boost the antibody response. The IACUC used to approve protocols using CFA; however, in recent years such use had been denied because of the pain and irritation it caused the mice. The IACUC denies the investigator permission to use CFA. The investigator appeals, arguing that she has just arrived from an institution which allows the use of CFA and has years of data using the adjuvant. She maintains that she must continue its use so that she is able to make valid comparisons between her old and new studies. How would you respond?

5.10 Your have just obtained your Ph.D. and been offered a postdoctoral position in the laboratory of Dr. Fremont. Upon arriving, you are somewhat dismayed to find the furious pace set by the other post-doctorals. They are not so much unfriendly as they are hard-driving. You have a bit of trouble getting settled and finding your niche. You haven't had a project assigned, so for a few days you have a chance to look around the lab. You are somewhat shocked at the way the monkeys are being treated—with nowhere near the level of care you have been trained to provide. You observe one student who is actually smoking during a surgical procedure. A second student drops a forceps on the floor, picks it up, and continues to use it in the surgical procedure. A third is working on a monkey who appears to have been severely injured, but the student tells you that he doesn't want to have to wait for another monkey. You finally say something when you see a fellow postdoctoral suturing an incision on an inadequately anesthetized monkey. "You're hurting him!" you yell, halfway angry and halfway stunned. The postdoctoral looks at you for a few seconds and continues suturing. The next day you receive your research project from the senior postdoctoral (Dr. Fremont is in Europe), and you bring up several of the incidents that you have witnessed. The senior post-doctoral acknowledges that an occasional corner may be cut, but says that there is no reason for concern. It's a high-pressure lab and people come there to get results. She reminds you that you will have your six-month review with Dr. Fremont "before you know it" and that if you plan to do a second year there, you had "better get cracking because Dr. Fremont only keeps the winners." What should you do?

Suggested Readings

In a chapter of this length, it has not been possible to consider all aspects of this complicated issue. For example, we have not placed the modern animal rights movement in the proper political context with other modern movements. The animal rights movement finds itself alternately in agreement and at odds with the environmental movement, the right to life movement, and various areas of feminist political and philosophical thought. Additionally, no mention has been made of the use of illegal actions such as laboratory break-ins, arson, violence, and threats of violence by some members of the animal rights movement. The following annotated list will help the student locate additional material for in-depth reading on these and other issues related to the use of animals in biomedical experimentation.

Rowan, A. N. 1984. *Of Mice, Models, and Men: A Critical Evaluation of Animal Research.* State University of New York Press, Albany, NY, p. 1–323. A good overview written by Andrew Rowan, a biochemist, former staffer at the Human Society of the United States, and current director of the Center for Animals and Public Policy at Tufts University School of Veterinary Medicine. Rowan is neither an abolitionist nor an advocate for all animal research. His book covers the history, attitudes, and treatment of animals used in both research and education.

Orlans, F. B. 1993. *In the Name of Science.* Oxford University Press, Oxford, p. 1–297. Another middle-of-the-road book. Orlans is on the faculty of the Kennedy Institute of Ethics at Georgetown University and is a former animal researcher at the National Institutes of Health. In addition to outlining the current political status of both animal rights and proresearch groups, she devotes chapters to the consideration of the workings of the IACUC, measurement of animal pain, and the controversial area of determining which species are capable of feeling pain.

Singer, P. 1990. *Animal Liberation,* 2nd ed. Avon Books, New York. Still considered by many as the "bible" of the animal rights movement. Even those activists who consider Singer's position too moderate continue to use the book to win new converts for the cause. Singer combines easy-to-read philosophy with arguments for vegetarianism and critiques of animal research and factory farming.

Regan, T. 1983. *The Case for Animal Rights.* University of California Press, Berkeley, CA, p. 1–425. Heavy on philosophy and difficult to read. Nevertheless, the book is important because most who call themselves "animal rights activists" embrace a philosophy much more like Regan's than Singer's.

Rollin, B. 1992. *Animal Rights and Human Morality.* Prometheus Books, Buffalo, NY, p. 1–248. Easy to read and more moderate in its view than the books of Singer and Regan. Rollin seems to hope for the cessation of animal use in research, while realizing that a more attainable goal is to improve the treatment of those animals which will be used in research for the foreseeable future.

Rachels, J. 1990. *Created from Animals: The Moral Implications of Darwinism.* Oxford University Press, Oxford. Rachels argues that the Darwinian revolution which transformed our traditional view of biology should similarly alter our view of morality and the role which animals have played within it.

Regan, T., and P. Singer. 1989. *Animal Rights and Human Obligations.* Prentice-Hall, Englewood Cliffs, NJ, p. 1–280. A book of short essays containing both historical and contemporary views of writers who support, or oppose, rights for animals.

Singer, P. 1985. *In Defense of Animals.* Perennial Library, New York, p. 1–224. Contains a number of contemporary essays in support of animal rights.

Leahy, M. P. T. 1991. *Against Liberation: Putting Animals in Perspective.* Routledge, New York. This British philosopher views the ethical direction taken by the animal rights philosophers as incorrect and argues for a more traditional moral view of animals. Leahy critiques positions taken by Singer, Regan, and other animal rights philosophers.

Carruthers, P. 1992. *The Animals Issue: Moral Theory in Practice.* Cambridge University Press, Cambridge. The University of Sheffield philosophy professor argues that while most books published recently seem to support the notion of rights for animals, this is not because this represents a consensus view among philosophers. As well as criticizing the position of the major animal rights philosophers, Carruthers describes a contractualist ethic which demands humane treatment for animals but does not grant them rights.

Sharpe, R. 1988. *The Cruel Deception: The Use of Animals in Medical Research.* Thorsons Publishing Group, Wellingborough, England, p. 1–288. Maintains that animal research has contributed little to human health, and that it is generally invalid because its results are not applicable to humans.

Paton, W. 1993. *Man and Mouse: Animals in Medical Research.* Oxford University Press, Oxford, p. 1–288. A defense of the scientific validity and utility of animal research.

Griffin, D. R. 1992. *Animal Minds.* The University of Chicago Press, Chicago, p. 1–310. Discussions of consciousness and thinking in animals.

Dawkins, M. S. 1980. *Animal Suffering: The Science of Animal Welfare.* Chapman and Hall, London, p. 1–149. Discussions of pain and suffering in animals.

Rollin, B. E. 1989. *The Unheeded Cry: Animal Consciousness, Animal Pain, and Science.* Oxford University Press, New York. Discussions of consciousness, pain, and suffering. Easy to read.

Newkirk, I. 1990. *Save the Animals: 101 Easy Things You Can Do.* Warner Books, New York, p. 1–192. An introduction to animal rights activism written by the director of PETA.

1990. *The Animal Rights Handbook: Everyday Ways to Save Animal Lives.* Living Planet Press, Venice, CA, p. 1–113. An introduction to animal rights activism.

Guillermo, K. S. 1993. *Monkey Business.* National Press Books, Washington, D.C., p. 1–254. PETA's view of the "Silver Spring Monkeys Case" which elevated the group to national prominence.

Newkirk, I. 1992. *Free the Animals!: The Untold Story of the U.S. Animal Liberation Front and Its Founder, Valerie.* The Noble Press, Inc., Chicago, p. 1–372. PETA's cofounder and national director writes about the Animal Liberation Front, a group which claims responsibility for numerous laboratory break-ins and terrorist acts.

Wolf, S. 1991. *A Declaration of War: Killing People to Save Animals and the Environment.* Patrick Henry Press, Grass Valley, CA, p. 1–119. A very strange book by the pseudonymous author Screaming Wolf. The publishers claim that the manuscript was delivered on a computer disk to two animal rights activists, who do not claim to support its call to violence, yet chose to publish the manuscript for "informational" purposes.

Scarce, R. 1990. *Eco-Warriors: Understanding the Radical Environmental Movement.* The Noble Press, Inc., Chicago, p. 1–291. A journalist attempts to place the animal rights movement into the context of radical environmentalism.

Jasper, J. M., and D. Nelkin. 1992. *The Animal Rights Crusade.* The Free Press, New York, p. 1–214. An examination of the movement by sociologists.

Sperling, S. 1988. *Animal Liberators: Research and Morality.* University of California Press, Berkeley, CA, p. 1–247. An anthropologist examines the animal rights movement in the light of its Victorian predecessors, feminism, and other contemporary movements in an extremely interesting and thought-provoking book.

REFERENCES

1. 1966. Concentration camps for dogs. *Life* **60(5),** February 4, p. 22–29.
2. 1985. *Guide for the Care and Use of Laboratory Animals.* NIH Publication No. 86-23. National Institutes of Health, Bethesda, MD.
3. 1986. *Public Health Service Policy on the Humane Care and Use of Laboratory Animals.* Office for Protection from Research Risks, National Institutes of Health, Bethesda, MD.
4. 1991. *Education and Training in the Care and Use of Laboratory Animals: A Guide for Developing Institutional Programs.* National Academy Press, Washington, D.C.
5. Arluke, A. 1990. Uneasiness among laboratory technicians. *Lab. Anim.* **19(4):**20–38.
6. Arluke, A. 1992. Trapped in a guilt cage. *New Sci.* **134:**33–35.
7. Arluke, A. 1993. Going into the closet with science. *J. Contemp. Ethnography* **20(3):**306–330.
8. Burd, S. 1993. U.S. Judge's ruling sets up new battle over care of lab animals. *Chron. Higher Educ.* March 10:A30.
9. Carruthers, P. 1992. *The Animals Issue: Moral Theory in Practice.* Cambridge University Press, Cambridge.
10. Cohen, C. 1986. The case for the use of animals in biomedical research. *N. Engl. J. Med.* **315(14):**865–870.
11. Dresser, R. 1988. Assessing harm and justification in animal research: federal policy opens the laboratory door. *Rutgers Law Rev.* **40(3):**723–796.
12. Elliot, C. 1992. Where ethics come from and what to do about it. *Hastings Center Rep.* **22(4):**28–35.
13. Elston, M. A. 1992. Victorian values and animal rights. *New Sci.* **134(1822):** 28–31.
14. Francione, G. L. 1987. Experimentation and the marketplace theory of the first amendment. *Univ. Penn. Law Rev.* **136(2):**417–512.
15. Francione, G. L. 1988. The constitutional status of restrictions on experiments involving nonhuman animals: a comment on Professor Dresser's analysis. *Rutgers Law Rev.* **40(3):**797–818.
16. Francione, G. L. 1990. Xenografts and animal rights. *Transplant. Proc.* **22(3):** 1044–1046.
17. French, R. D. 1975. The mind of antivivisection: medicine, p. 288–344. *In Antivivisection and Medical Science in Victorian Society.* Princeton University Press, Princeton, NJ.
18. French, R. D. 1975. Anatomy of an agitation, p. 220–287. *In Antivivisection and Medical Science in Victorian Society.* Princeton University Press, Princeton, NJ.
19. Frey, R. G. 1980. *Interests and Rights: The Case Against Animals.* Oxford Clarendon Press, Oxford.

20. **Frey, R. G.** 1983. *Rights, Killing, and Suffering: Moral Vegetarianism and Applied Ethics.* Blackwell, Oxford.
21. **Frey, R. G.** 1989. The case against animal rights, p. 115–118. *In* T. Regan and P. Singer (eds.), *Animal Rights and Human Obligations.* Prentice-Hall, Englewood Cliffs, NJ.
22. **Frey, R. G., and W. Paton.** 1989. Vivisection, morals, and medicine: an exchange, p. 223–236. *In* T. Regan and P. Singer (eds.), *Animal Rights and Human Obligations.* Prentice-Hall, Englewood Cliffs, NJ.
23. **Herzog, H.** 1990. Philosophy, ethology, and animal rights. *Trends* June/July:14–17.
24. **Herzog, H.** 1994. Human morality and animal research: confessions and quandaries. *Am. Scholar* Summer:337–349.
25. **Herzog, H. A.** 1988. The moral status of mice. *Am. Psychol.* **43**:473–474.
26. **Herzog, H. A.** 1990. Discussing animal rights and animal research in the classroom. *Teach. Psychol.* **17(2)**:90–94.
27. **Herzog, H. A.** 1991. Conflicts of interests: kittens and boa constrictor, pets and research. *Am. Psychol.* **46**:246–248.
28. **Jamison, W. V., and W. M. Lunch.** 1992. Rights of animals, perceptions of science, and political activism: profile of American animal rights activists. *Sci. Technol. Hum. Values* **17(4)**:438–458.
29. **Leahy, M. P. T.** 1991. *Against Liberation: Putting Animals in Perspective.* Routledge, New York.
30. **Mann, M. D., D. A. Crouse, and E. D. Prentice.** 1991. Appropriate animal numbers in biomedical research in light of animal welfare concerns. *Lab. Anim. Sci.* **41(1)**:6–14.
31. **Mappes, T. A., and J. S. Zembaty.** 1991. Biomedical ethics and ethical theory, p. 1–44. *In* T. A. Mappes and J. S. Zembaty (eds.), *Biomedical Ethics.* McGraw-Hill, New York.
32. **Midgley, M.** 1989. Are you an animal?, p. 1–18. *In* G. Langley (ed.), *Animal Experimentation: The Consensus Changes.* Chapman and Hall, New York.
33. **Midgley, M.** 1989. The case for restricting research using animals, p. 216–222. *In* T. Regan and P. Singer (eds.), *Animal Rights and Human Obligations.* Prentice-Hall, Englewood Cliffs, NJ.
34. **Midgley, M.** 1992. The mixed community, p. 211–225. *In* E. C. Hargrove (ed.), *The Animal Rights/Environmental Ethics Debate: The Environmental Perspective.* State University of New York Press, Albany, NY.
35. **Midgley, M.** 1992. The significance of species, p. 121–136. *In* E. C. Hargrove (ed.), *The Animal Rights/Environmental Ethics Debate: The Environmental Perspective.* State University of New York Press, Albany, NY.
36. **Orlans, F. B.** 1993. *In the Name of Science*, p. 1–297. Oxford University Press, Oxford.
37. **Porter, D. G.** 1992. Ethical scores for animal experiments. *Nature* **356**:101–102.
38. **Post, S. G.** 1993. The emergence of species impartiality: a medical critique of biocentrism. *Perspect. Biol. Med.* **36**:289–300.
39. **Regan, T.** 1983. *The Case for Animal Rights*, p. 1–425. University of California Press, Berkeley, CA.

40. **Regan, T.** 1985. The case for animal rights, p. 13–26. *In* P. Singer (ed.), *In Defence of Animals*. Basil Blackwell, Oxford.
41. **Rowan, A. N.** 1984. *Of Mice, Models, and Men: A Critical Evaluation of Animal Research*, p. 1–323. State University of New York Press, Albany, NY.
42. **Russell, W. M. S., and R. L. Burch.** 1959. *Principles of Humane Animal Experimentation*, p. 1–238. Charles C Thomas, Springfield, IL.
43. **Singer, P.** 1986. All animals are equal, p. 215–227. *In* P. Singer (ed.), *Applied Ethics*. Oxford University Press, Oxford.
44. **Singer, P.** 1990. Tools for research, p. 25–94. *In Animal Liberation*, 2nd ed. Avon Books, New York.
45. **Singer, P.** 1990. All animals are equal, p. 1–23. *In Animal Liberation*, 2nd ed. Avon Books, New York.
46. **Singer, P.** 1990. *Animal Liberation*, 2nd ed. Avon Books, New York.
47. **Sperling, S.** 1988. Humans, animals and machines, p. 131–155. *In Animal Liberators: Research and Morality*. University of California Press, Berkeley, CA.
48. **Sperling, S.** 1988. The Victorian antivivisection movement, p. 25–48. *In Animal Liberators: Research and Morality*. University of California Press, Berkeley, CA.
49. **Sperling, S.** 1988. Natural incursions, p. 51–75. *In Animal Liberators: Research and Morality*. University of California Press, Berkeley, CA.
50. **United States District Court for the District of Columbia.** 1992. Civil Action No. 90-1872 (CRR). Filed January 8, 1992. Animal Legal Defense Fund *et al.*, Plaintiffs, v. Edward R. Madigan, *et al.*, Defendants. Opinion of Charles R. Richey, United States District Judge.
51. **United States District Court for the District of Columbia.** 1993. Civil Action No. 91-1328 (CRR). Filed February 25, 1993. Animal Legal Defense Fund *et al.*, Plaintiffs, v. USDA Secretary Espy *et al.*, Defendants. Opinion of Charles R. Richey, United States District Judge.

6 | Use of Humans in Biomedical Experimentation

Paul S. Swerdlow

Overview

There are many important ethical issues in scientific endeavors, but none has been better codified than experimentation involving human beings as subjects. Much of early medicine undoubtedly involved experimentation, most of which was not regulated. In fact, the rules for experimentation with people were initially summarized in the Nuremberg Principles that came out of the Nuremberg trials at the end of World War II. These trials held accountable those involved in human experimentation performed without the consent of the subjects.

Unfortunately, a significant number of ethically questionable studies have been performed (2), before and after promulgation of the Nuremberg Principles. A particularly egregious example is the Tuskegee study conducted at the Tuskegee Institute with funding from the U.S. Public Health Service (6). The aim of the 1932 study was to determine the course of untreated syphilis in African Americans, a disease that was widely believed to be a distinct entity from that in Caucasians. The arsenic- and mercury-based therapy then in use was quite toxic but generally believed to be beneficial. No patient consent was obtained in this study wherein spinal taps were disguised as "free treatment." Even the scientific basis was flawed since most of the 412 infected men had received some initial treatment as an inducement to participate in the study. It was later decided that, since their treatment had been inadequate, follow-up as an untreated cohort was warranted. The study clearly documented a 20% decrease in life span for those infected as compared with the control group of 204 uninfected men.

In the 1940s, when penicillin was found to be effective therapy, the study was nonetheless continued. It was reasoned that this was the last chance to study untreated syphilis because of soon to be widespread antibiotic use. Patients were not informed about the potential new therapy, although their infections could have been cured by penicillin. As late as 1969, a review panel allowed the study to continue. The Macon County Medical Society, which included African American physicians, promised to assist in the study and to refer all patients before using antibiotics for *any* reason. In 1972 the study was finally reported in the public press. In 1973, more than 20 years after penicillin was in widespread use, the government finally took steps to ensure treatment of the few surviving infected patients.

The World Medical Association has sponsored two conferences in Helsinki to formalize guiding principles for the ethical use of humans in biomedical experimentation. These are known as the Conference of Helsinki (1964) and Helsinki II (1975). The text of the Helsinki II proclamation is reprinted at the end of this chapter.

The Issue of Informed Consent

Key among the principles of experimentation on human subjects is the concept of informed consent. Several elements are required for informed consent. The person must first be "competent to consent"— to understand consequences and to make decisions. The decisions do not have to meet any particular criteria for "good" decisions—he or she may enter a study for the "wrong" reason or may make a decision someone else thinks is "bad." In other words, one must simply need to be able to understand the consequences of various decisions and have the capacity to make such a decision. In practice, many people who are clearly competent routinely make bad decisions regarding relationships, employment, medical care, and many other matters. The standard of competence for medical research is no different.

Consent must also be voluntary, that is, free from coercion. Coercion to participate in studies, however, can be very subtle and at the same time powerful. Coercion can come from many sources, including the patient's family, the researcher, the physician, the institution, and even the health care system itself. While most researchers and institutions avoid coercing study participants, subtle coercions may not be apparent to those conducting the research, let alone the potential subjects for the research. Some of these elements are difficult to control. Family coercion to participate in some form of therapy is often strong, even when no clear benefit exists. This is often seen in cancer chemotherapy where, even though prolongation of survival may be minimal and treatment fraught with side effects, family pressure to take treatment can nevertheless be intense. This is usually related to standard therapy, but the same factors may pertain in research situations.

Similarly, coercion can become part of the health care system. In situations where no standard therapy exists, experimental therapies may be the only alternative. In aggressive attempts to control costs, health insurance plans are limiting the physician's freedom to embark on untested therapies by calling them "experimental." Most health care policies do not cover experimental expenses, and an ethical dilemma arises where all potential therapies for the disease in question are experimental. The result may be that, in the near future, only those willing to enroll in well-designed clinical trials will be allowed to receive experimental therapies. These trials often compare the experimental therapy with existing therapy or with no therapy at all. The patient may have to choose between the study and a chance of therapy or no therapy. Such situations must be closely scrutinized for coercion.

Coercion by the basic researcher (one not licensed to treat patients), physician, or the institution can also come into play and must be controlled. Researchers are often reimbursed in clinical studies on a per-patient basis. The per-patient fee covers the experimental costs, and often a portion of the researcher's salary and even the departmental budget as well. There is thus great incentive to enroll as many patients as possible. While the basic researcher usually has little to use to coerce people into participating (other than reimbursement for the activity), a physician-researcher has much more power. This power is likely to increase with new changes anticipated in the U.S. health care system. Currently, the physician to a large extent controls the patient's access to that system, and is often totally entrusted to make medical decisions for the patient. Many patients refuse to even question their physicians regarding these decisions, in part because they trust them because they possess requisite specialized knowledge and in part because of paternalistic (or maternalistic) attitudes held by many physicians. Under such circumstances, it is easy for patients to feel that if they decline to participate in a study, they may lose a precious doctor–patient relationship and even access to the health care system. Such issues must be addressed through consent forms and patient education or coercion may occur. This is especially likely if the physician is a participant in or will benefit from the research (e.g., the research is conducted by the department employing the physician). It is also important to regard the circumstances of the study and how the study will be employed in special populations where coercion is more likely (see below).

Consent must also be informed. The participant must have adequate information to make a valid decision. The participant has the right to hear about all known risks of the study, including risks even beyond what would normally be discussed for medical informed consent. When routinely informing a patient about potential risks of a procedure or course of treatment, the physician makes an effort to present all realistic risks that are likely to affect the decisionmaking of the patient. However, known risks of extremely small magnitude are often not mentioned. They are confusing and may adversely affect decisionmaking to the detriment of the patient. For example, risks that are significantly less likely than the risk of dying in a car accident on the way to the doctor's office are often not disclosed. With a study, however, particularly one that is not of therapeutic intent, all known risks should be disclosed for truly informed consent.

Merely presenting the information is not sufficient. Informed consent requires comprehension of the risks by the participant. There should be a test to verify that the person really understands the various options and risks and potential benefits of the study. For this reason, many institutions encourage that the witness to the signature on the consent form be a relative or friend of the participant. This provides another person who hears the same information and may ask additional questions and can ensure that the concepts were presented in an understandable way.

Who must ensure that the above obligations are fulfilled? It is the obligation of all who participate in the research to ensure that informed consent is obtained. This duty is not restricted to those who obtain the informed consent or to those involved solely with the clinical parts of the study. It is an obligation of all involved. It can be delegated to parts of the group but cannot be delegated lightly; that is, all involved are responsible to see that it is done correctly. It is essential for all involved to read the consent form and then ensure that the study, its risks, and its benefits are fairly and understandably presented.

Institutional Review Boards

Institutions receiving federal support in the United States are required to have an Institutional Review Board (IRB) to approve and oversee research on human subjects. Similar committees are found in other countries, but the rules and composition of these vary (10). The rules on the formation of U.S. committees are quite easy to comply with and most academic institutions have larger committees than required. The committee must include at least five members and the membership list must be filed with the U.S. Secretary of Health and Human Services. All five members cannot have the same profession and there must be at least one member with primary concerns in nonscientific areas (often a lawyer, ethicist, or clergyman). There must also be at least one member not affiliated with the institution nor with family so affiliated. The nonaffiliated member may also be the nonscientific member.

Approval of projects requires a simple majority vote. At least one nonscientific member of the committee must vote, but does not have to vote for approval. No member is allowed to participate in the review of a project in which he or she has a personal interest. The committee may invite experts to appear, but such experts may not vote. Proposals must be rereviewed yearly, and there must be written procedures which prescribe the operations of the committee. Serious or continuing noncompliance with the process must be reported to the Secretary of Health and Human Services.

The committee is charged with specific criteria by which to review proposals. First the risks to subjects must be minimized consistent with the aims of the research. Ideally, proposed procedures would be those already being performed for diagnostic or therapeutic purposes. For research to be ethically valid, it must first be technically valid. Even a study with minimal risk requires that valid scientific results be obtained or it cannot be justified. This is most often a problem with small clinical studies where statistically valid data may be difficult to obtain. Common reasons for such small studies include:

- *Study of a rare disease or disorder.* These are often called "orphan diseases" and are commonly ignored by pharmaceutical companies. The small potential market often cannot justify the drug development costs. The Food and Drug Administration, however, periodically sponsors studies of drugs for orphan diseases.

- *Pilot studies of new therapies.* It is often difficult to get funding for large and therefore expensive clinical studies. Pilot studies test feasibility of new treatments but are generally not sufficient to establish efficacy. They provide the information needed to properly design and obtain funding for the larger study.

These types of studies must have clearly defined endpoints so the IRB can determine their risk-to-benefit ratio. Valid endpoints can include determination of treatment toxicity, patient compliance, or drug pharmacokinetics. Attempting to determine efficacy of treatments with too few patients, however, will likely create problems at the IRB. Statistician members in particular will instantly realize that the chances of determining efficacy with a small population are nil unless dramatic changes are found in easily measured outcomes. A good statistical analysis is often essential for proper study design and can save time and unnecessary effort with the IRB, with granting agencies, and subsequently with data analysis.

Most importantly, the risks to subjects must be reasonable in relation to anticipated benefits. Study benefits include benefits to the research subject as well as the importance of the knowledge that may reasonably be expected to result. In assessing the risk / benefit ratio of the project, only the risks and benefits of the research should be considered. Risks of procedures that would still be performed if not in the study should not be considered. Similarly a beneficial procedure performed as part of a study cannot be considered a benefit if the same procedure would be performed without the study.

For clinical studies where two different treatments are being compared, there must be a valid null hypothesis that the two arms are equivalent. This is the concept of equipoise, that neither of the two treatments is known to be better. The researcher should be able to honestly say that there is no convincing data that one arm is better. If one arm is known to be better, the point of the study is moot and the research is no longer ethical. This includes placebo studies where the test treatment is compared to no treatment at all. Such studies may be reasonable if the efficacy of the treatment being tested is not known and there is no known efficacious therapy.

The committee is prohibited from considering long-range effects of research on public policy that may result from the research. For example, in reviewing a study of an expensive therapy for dissolution of gallstones, the committee should not take into account the potential bankrupting of the health care system if the procedure were eventually used on all gallstone patients.

Selection of subjects must be equitable. For example, it is not appropriate to restrict a study to people with health insurance in the hopes that such patients will eventually financially support the hospital should they return to have other medical problems treated. There is also a national effort to ensure that minority populations and women are not excluded from studies as has been done in the past. One reason often used in the past to exclude women from studies was the issue of pregnancy. A new drug has likely not been tested in human pregnancy and will pose an unknown risk to such pregnancies. It was often felt simpler not to include women so as not to have to worry about pregnancy. Currently, most studies will allow women using medically approved birth control to participate.

The Institutional Review Board and the Informed Consent Issue

IRBs must ensure that informed consent is sought from each prospective subject or his / her legally authorized representative. Those unable to consent but who have an appropriate legal representative or guardian may participate if such representative gives informed consent. All consents must be documented and signed by a witness. It is important that the witness not be part of the investigating team to avoid questions of conflict of interest. The best witness is a friend or relative of the participant. Such a person often has a background similar to the participant's and can help ensure that the study is explained in terms they can both understand. In addition, he or she will be able to ask questions and sometimes even help explain the study to the participant.

The research must make adequate provision for monitoring data to ensure the safety of subjects. Such information is also required by the Food Drug Administration for new agents. Adequate provisions must be made as well to protect privacy. Records containing identifying information should be maintained in locked locations and restricted to those who have a need to use the information and who are trained in medical confidentiality or privacy. It is especially important not to discuss such information in public places such as hallways, elevators, or lunchrooms where comments might be overheard. It is often a good idea to create a second database lacking identifying information for ease of use and convenience.

Special provisions must be made for studies where some or all of the subjects are likely to be vulnerable to coercion or undue influence. This includes people with acute or severe physical or mental illness and those who are economically or educationally disadvantaged. One such safeguard could be a patient representative to ensure that, where studies are complicated and involve acute medical situations, or include people with limited education, subjects completely understand all implications. Consent forms must be read to those who cannot read or read well and should be written so they are easy to understand. It often helps to have the consent reviewed by those used to dealing with the educationally disadvantaged.

There is an increasing trend for consents to be approved by central authorities for large projects involving substantial numbers of people. While this may seem intrusive, such efforts have so far yielded high-quality consent forms by employing people with expertise in the creation of such forms and who are skilled in presenting complex topics in lay language. With large double-blind studies, a separate data and safety monitoring committee is often used.

Certain types of research are exempt from consent requirements by the federal government and most IRBs. Consent is not needed for research conducted in educational settings involving normal educational practices. This includes research on education instructional strategies, the efficacy or the comparison of instructional techniques, or curricula or classroom management methods. Research involving the use of educational tests (cognitive, diagnostic, aptitude, achievement) is also exempt if the information taken from these sources is recorded in such a manner that subjects cannot be identified directly or indirectly.

Research involving survey, interviews, or observation of public behavior does not need consent unless responses are recorded in such a manner that the subjects can be identified directly or indirectly, where the responses or behaviors could place the subject at risk for criminal or civil liability, and where the research deals with sensitive aspects of behavior such as illegal conduct, drug use, or sexual behavior. Research involving surveys or interviews is also exempt from consents when respondents are public officials or candidates for public office.

What should be included in an informed consent? Consent forms fulfill several roles in human research. They are designed to describe the study in detail, including risks and benefits. They can, however, also be a contract and include compensation for participation in the study. Consents must spell out the participants' rights, including the right to withdraw from the study at any time. They must also reassure participants that they will not forfeit any other rights because of refusal to participate or withdrawal from the study. The form should specify what happens if a participant becomes pregnant and whether birth control is required to participate. The consent also provides the participant with the phone number of the investigator and for the IRB, should a participant with concerns not wish to speak with the investigator. Each institution has its own format, but uniformity of protocol and consent formats aids in the review process.

The Institutional Review Board and Expedited Review

Many committees have procedures for expedited review for specific types of research involving no more than minimal risk. These include procedures listed below, adapted from the *Code of Federal Regulations* (45 C.F.R. 46).

Collection of:

Cells or substances from the body that are easily and nontraumatically obtained such as hair, nail clippings, surface skin by gentle scraping, excreta, sweat, saliva (not via cannulation of salivary duct), amniotic fluid at time of rupture of membranes, deciduous teeth, or dental plaque all if collected in nondisfiguring, nontraumatic manner.

Permanent teeth if extraction needed anyway; placenta after delivery.

Blood by venipuncture in amounts not exceeding 450 ml every 8 weeks and no more than twice weekly from normal volunteers over 18 and not pregnant.

Study of existing data or specimens.

Recording of data from:
   Procedures routinely employed in clinical practice (pulse, blood pressure, respiration rate, temperature, weight, sensory acuity testing, EKG, EEG, thermography, sonigrams, but excluding studies requiring exposure to radiation (X-rays or microwaves). Moderate exercise by healthy volunteers.
   Research on behavior or individual characteristics including perception, cognition, game theory, or test development provided the study does not manipulate subject's behavior or cause stress to subjects.

Human Experimentation Involving Special Populations

Incompetent patients

It is often assumed that those with mental illness or who are not able to provide informed consent must be excluded from all studies. This is not the case. Consent must be provided by the legally responsible person, and the study must be designed in such a way that adequate safeguards exist for the participants. It would seem unfair to deprive these people of the right to participate in potentially therapeutic studies or to prevent information from being gathered to help people with mental disorders. Clearly, the IRB and the researchers must ensure that individual rights are respected. They must also take into account that participation in arduous programs without being able to understand the reason for the treatments makes such programs much more difficult to endure. This type of research may therefore be inappropriate for certain populations (certain chemotherapy trials, for example). Psychiatric patients may be particularly vulnerable emotionally. Particular attention must be paid to avoiding covert (and likely unintentional) coercion. Furthermore, it has been suggested that research personnel should use the medical definitions of informed consent for certain studies in this patient population rather than the more comprehensive information usually required (4) in an effort to reduce patient anxiety. Thus, the IRB has special responsibilities for protocols involving these patients.

Prisoners

Prisoners constitute an excellent example of a population that requires additional safeguards for consent for scientific study. The nature of incarceration affords numerous potential coercions, and thus federal regulations specifically offer additional safeguards for this population (46 C.F.R. 45). Only certain types of federally sponsored research can be performed on prisoners. These include:

- Study of possible causes, effects, and processes of incarceration or criminal behavior that present no more than minimal risk or inconvenience to the prisoner.
- Studies of prisons as institutional structures or of prisoners as incarcerated persons.
- Research on conditions affecting prisoners as a class such as vaccine studies on hepatitis due to the increased incidence of hepatitis in prisons, or social or psychological problems such as alcoholism or drug addiction. The Secretary of Health and Human Services must consult with experts in penology, medicine, and ethics and give notice in the *Federal Register* of intent to approve such research.
- Research on both innovative and accepted practices which have the intent to improve the health or well-being of the subject. If control groups will be used in the protocol, the Secretary must again consult with experts and give notice as above.

There are very specific requirements for the IRB, including that a prisoner or a prisoner representative must be a member of the IRB. A prisoner representative must have the appropriate background and experience to serve as a true representative of the prisoners. Another requirement is that a majority of the IRB (exclusive of prisoner members) must have no association with the prisons involved. There is no requirement that the prisoner or prisoner representative must vote for a given proposal for it to be enacted.

The IRB must further determine that any advantages gained by the prisoner by participating are not of such a magnitude that the prisoner's ability to weigh the risks of participation are impaired. These would include advantages in living conditions, medical care, quality of food, amenities, potential earnings, and outside contacts. The risks involved must also be risks that would be accepted by non-prisoner volunteers. Study information must be presented in an understandable manner for the population.

Selection of subjects in prison must be fair to all prisoners and cannot be arbitrarily used or influenced by prisoners or prison authorities. Studies must not be used as a reward or method to control the inmate population.

Contrary to public impression, participation in scientific or medical studies cannot be taken into account by parole boards in determining eligibility for parole. The prisoner must be specifically informed that parole will not be affected. Allowing participation to affect parole would be a good example of undue influence or coercion to participate.

Where follow-up is required, arrangements must be made for the varying lengths of sentence of the prisoners. The researchers should also consider the likelihood of noncompliance after the sentence is over. The potential import of these arrangements is illustrated by the tragic case of a 35-year-old prisoner who developed testicular cancer while incarcerated. The prisoner was placed on a standard, noninvestigational therapy with his consent. With aggressive chemotherapy, testicular cancer is largely curable. After the first course of chemotherapy obtained a good response, the court, at the county's request, paroled the prisoner. The reason for parole was not made clear to the medical staff, but suspicions were that either it was a compassionate parole (which seemed strange for a largely curable, as opposed to terminal, cancer) or that the county did not wish to pay the costly medical bills for the therapy. The prisoner, who had tolerated the chemotherapy well, left the hospital against medical advice in the middle of a treatment saying he had "things to do." He never returned for the needed therapy and was lost to follow-up. While it was clearly his right to leave, it is also likely that the cancer recurred. Recurrent cancer has a diminished prognosis and if left untreated would undoubtedly be fatal. If the prisoner had been on a study, it is certain he would not have continued with it. In this particular case, some of the medical staff felt that the county, by paroling the prisoner, had converted his sentence to a death sentence (albeit with the prisoner's unintentional collaboration).

Children

For children under the age of 18 years, consent must be given by the parents or guardians. For research that involves significant risk, both parents must consent when available unless only one parent has legal responsibility or custody. In addition, assent or agreement of the child is required where the IRB deems that he or she is capable. In making this determination, the IRB must consider the age, maturity, and psychological state of the children involved. This can be done for all children involved in a given protocol or individually. If the IRB determines that the capability of the child is too limited or if the research may offer benefits important to the health or well-being of the child, assent is not required.

Recently, it has been pointed out that certain behaviors commonly accepted in society put children at much greater risk than do most research studies. G. Koren *et al.* calculated the risk of a babysitter having to deal with a severe medical emergency in Canada (7). They calculated that each year at least 900 Canadian babysitters would have to deal with an acute asthmatic attack in one of their charges and that 26 would likely have a child who experiences sudden infant death syndrome (SIDS) while under their care. These situations would place the babysitters, often between ages 10 and 15, at risk of emotional trauma far greater than would most research studies. The authors argue that if a child is deemed mature enough to supervise younger children in potentially extremely dangerous situations, he or she is likely to be able to fully consent to most research studies.

Children who are wards of the state or any other agency can be included in research only if the research is either related to their status as wards or conducted in institutions in which the majority of children involved are not wards. In such cases, the IRB shall require appointment of an advocate—not associated with the research, the investigator, or the guardian organization—who agrees to act in the best interests of the child for the duration of the child's participation in the research.

Additional restrictions are imposed for research with greater than minimal risk. However, where there is greater than minimal risk but also the possibility of direct benefit to the child, the IRB must determine that the risk is justified by the anticipated benefits. The risk/benefit ratio must also be at least as good as all alternative approaches. Where there is no prospect of direct benefit, but the research is likely to yield important knowledge about a disorder, the risk must represent a minor increase over minimal risks. The interventions must be comparable to those inherent in the actual or expected medical, dental, social, or educational situations. The information to be obtained must be of vital import for the understanding or amelioration of the subject's disorder or condition. To bypass these restrictions, there must be a reasonable opportunity to achieve further understanding, prevention, or alleviation of a serious problem affecting the health or welfare of children. Nevertheless, the Secretary of Health and Human Services must consult with a panel of experts, and ensure that such a condition exists and that the research will be ethically conducted.

These restrictions may seem excessive and may indeed slow research in some areas. It must be remembered, however, that for children who are not old enough to assent, the parents and the IRB remain their sole advocates. There is even some indication that parents who volunteer their children for studies may be psychologically different from those who don't, making the issue of study regulation and control even more important (5).

Fetal Tissue Research

There has been a great deal of controversy surrounding the use of fetal tissues in research, specifically in transplantation of fetal tissue (3, 11). During the administrations of Ronald Reagan and George Bush, all federal funding was discontinued for research on transplantation of fetal tissues, largely out of concern that funding might encourage abortion. On February 1, 1993, the Secretary of Health and Human Services ended the moratorium on funding of fetal research. Criteria have now been promulgated by multiple sources regarding the conduct of fetal research and fall into several categories.

It is believed important to separate the abortion from the research. This includes issues such as the decision to terminate a pregnancy, the timing of the abortion, and which abortion procedures to use. Payments and other inducements to participate in research on fetal tissues are prohibited. Directed donations are prohibited, including the use of related fetal tissue transplants. Anonymity between donor and recipient must be maintained. The donor will not know who will receive the tissue, nor will the recipient or transplant team know the donor.

Consent of the pregnant woman is required and is sufficient unless the father objects (except in cases of incest or rape). The decision and consent to abort must precede discussion of the possible use of fetal tissue and any request for such consent that might be required for such use. Recipients of such tissues, researchers, and health care participants must also be properly informed about the source of the tissues in question.

The guidelines may well undergo continued revision. Some suggest that the person performing the abortion or any physician on the supply side of fetal tissue not be allowed to be a coauthor or receive support from the study. Others believe that the consent of the mother is not appropriate and that an external consent should be sought.

D. K. Martin argues that, contrary to NIH guidelines, it is unethical to withhold information on fetal tissue donation because it may be important information for women making the decision to abort (8). He also argues that in time women will know of the option anyway. Attempts to make the abortion decision in the absence of knowledge of tissue donation options will become futile as the information of such transplants is disseminated. It should be emphasized that this is currently a minority opinion.

Case Studies

6.1 A graduate student is doing a two-month rotation through a lab engaged in lymphocyte research. For this period of time, his grade is based solely on the evaluation by his lab mentor. He does not like needles. Is he really free to refuse to donate blood to the lab?

6.2 A prestigious medical institution with an active research program has determined that it will need to have all of its patients in a study in order to reach needed accrual for statistical purposes. It sets up a policy where all patients eligible for a protocol are to be treated on that protocol or referred to other institutions for care. Is this coercive? Is this policy acceptable at a public institution that provides care to people unable to go elsewhere for financial reasons?

6.3 One incentive often mentioned as a benefit of a clinical study is a free physical examination. This inducement is much stronger for those lacking medical insurance and access to the health care system. Is such an inducement coercive, as it appeals more to those with greater need? Alternatively, is it merely a good inducement likely to benefit the participant who cannot obtain an exam any other way?

6.4 Part of the evaluation of a National Cancer Institute-designated Comprehensive Cancer Center is an evaluation of the fraction of the patients seen who are placed on study protocols. The funding of such centers is a major source of income for academic divisions associated with cancer centers. Do such evaluations put too much emphasis on protocols? Are they likely to result in institution- and physician-based patient coercion? Some argue that properly designed protocols offer state-of-the-art established treatments as well as the most promising experimental therapies. Is this argument convincing to you?

6.5 You are sitting as a member of an institutional review board that examines proposals for the use of humans in medical experiments. A proposal currently under consideration would involve the administration to patients of fluorescently labeled, mouse-derived monoclonal antibodies. These immunologic reagents would be used in testing their ability to localize and diagnose tumors. A committee discussion ensues concerning the informed consent form proposed for use in these experiments. Specifically, one member of the committee argues that the consent form fails to reveal that participation in this study could preclude the future use of antitumor monoclonal antibody therapy in these patients. This argument is based on the potential of such patients to mount an anti-mouse antibody response. Considerable disagreement among the committee members erupts as a result of this issue. Comment on the appropriateness of including such a disclosure in the informed consent form.

6.6 A researcher wishes to study the metabolism of alveolar macrophages in patients with severe pneumonia and to correlate these findings with the clinical outcome of the patient. She proposes to take small samples of pulmonary lavage fluid to obtain the required cells. The fluid would be obtained only from those patients who would be undergoing pulmonary lavage for medical reasons. Pulmonary lavage is a standard medical procedure where a flexible fiber optic bronchoscope is passed into the lungs of a mildly sedated patient. Fluid is then used to wash out the contents of the alveoli in the lung and is then withdrawn. The procedure is used clinically to help diagnose difficult pulmonary problems. Does she need to include the risks of pulmonary lavage in the consent form? Does she need to worry that her pulmonologist collaborator will perform lavage on patients not needing the procedure to provide additional study samples?

6.7 An investigator wants to screen a recombinant bacteriophage library with antiserum to a specific protein made by a common human oral bacterium. Her initial intent is to raise polyclonal antibodies in rabbits by using the purified protein. However, following discussions with colleagues, the investigator learns that many adults produce antibodies to a number of proteins associated with this bacterium. Her colleague indicates that he has dozens of serum samples from individual patients stored in his freezer. He suggests that she pool these sera and use the pooled material to screen her library. Is this strategy appropriate in terms of proper use of human materials in research? What if any paperwork should be filed?

6.8 A 64-year-old man presents with advanced lung cancer. He has a long history of depression resulting in several suicide attempts and several hospitalizations for clinically severe depression. He often skips his antidepressant medications. There is no standard therapy that has been shown to statistically prolong life with his cancer, but some patients do seem to respond to aggressive chemotherapy and may live longer. An experimental protocol is available for a new therapy that has been tested in small trials and is now being compared with aggressive chemotherapy. The family (including his brother, who has been appointed his legal guardian) is most interested in treatment. The patient is clinically depressed and states he is not interested in therapy. His psychiatrist is concerned that this may be a subtle way of committing suicide. Should the researcher attempt to place the patient on study? This would require consent of the guardian and probably also a court ruling since the patient is opposed to the therapy. If not placed on study, should chemotherapy be given anyway? What would be the effect on the patient of chemotherapeutic complications given that the therapy is not wanted in the first place?

6.9 A physician's salary is partly dependent on his grant funding. Thus, if his grant funding decreases, so will his salary. He is running a drug company study which reimburses for costs and for salary on a per-patient basis. The physician decides to offer a small incentive to the other physicians in the medical center for referring patients who are good candidates for study. Is an incentive of a gift certificate for dinner (value $30) reasonable? Is it likely to result in patient coercion? What if the gift is a textbook worth $150, or $150 in cash?

6.10 You ask a fellow graduate student and her husband, whom you ran into in the hall, to donate 10 cc of blood each for one of your established protocols. While enumerating the T cell subsets, you find very low values in the husband. This is worrisome as AIDS can cause such low values. Do you tell him? Do you tell his wife? You ask your mentor what should be done. She says she will take care of the situation. Two days later you see the husband in your mentor's office and she later informs you that he was told. Two weeks later it becomes apparent that your fellow graduate student, the spouse of the man with the low T cell subsets, still doesn't know about the problem. Do you tell her?

6.11 Prior to the emergence of AIDS, a noted hematologist wished to study whether idiopathic thrombocytopenic purpura (ITP), a disease where the platelet count drops dangerously low despite increased platelet production, might be due to the presence of an autoantibody directed against the person's own platelets. He drew blood from one of these patients, isolated serum, which contains the antibodies in the blood, and injected the serum into his own vein. He then monitored his platelet count and documented an abrupt drop in his own platelet count. Indeed the count dropped so far that he had a nearly fatal bleed and required hospitalization. After recovery, he again drew blood from another patient and injected a smaller amount into his arm to document that antibodies existed in this patient as well. This time the platelet count did not drop as far and he did not bleed. Subsequently a paper was published documenting similar results from a larger number of patients whose serum was injected into an undisclosed number of volunteers. This information was a major contribution to the understanding of ITP. Is such research reasonable? Should it be regulated by the IRB? Is there self-coercion here? Is the researcher so committed to the science that there is no perspective on potential self-injury? Should researchers be allowed to experiment on themselves?

6.12   One of the best tissues for research study is blood. It is easily obtained and contains a considerable number of intact and already separated cells. Each 5 cc (one teaspoon) of blood from a normal individual contains about 2.5×10^{10} red blood cells, 2.5×10^7 white blood cells, and 1.5×10^9 platelets as well as over 300 mg of plasma proteins. Many labs are constantly seeking volunteers to donate blood, a simple and safe procedure. Can those involved in research, especially junior members of the lab, easily refuse to donate such samples? In some locations, IRBs sensitive to this issue have decided that those in a given lab cannot donate blood for that lab but can donate for other labs. It is believed that this would then allow them to refuse more readily. Is this reasonable? Should similar restrictions be considered for other study situations involving laboratory volunteers?

6.13   A technician working with platelets asks her supervisor if she can use her own blood as the normal control instead of using donated controls. She argues that this will allow her to work without gloves and to avoid any chance of infectious complications. The institutional IRB does not allow those in the lab to donate for the lab. Is her request reasonable? What would you do if you were her supervisor? She states that her husband would also be willing to donate. She would still like to work without gloves. Is this okay? Is the husband free to refuse?

6.14 A researcher wishes to study the utility of morphine maintenance in drug users. Morphine in pure form is relatively safe, certainly much safer than street drugs. Such a program might minimize the spread of AIDS in the drug-using population. Is any study of this sort ethical? If so, what sorts of ethical and review problems might have to be considered in such research? If not, why not? (See reference 9.)

6.15 A researcher has developed a new drug for malaria and wishes to test it in humans. Since there are too few cases in the United States, he wants to test it in Africa on a population at significant risk for malaria. Unfortunately, the drug is quite expensive to manufacture and is unlikely to be made available to the population of the country chosen for testing. Is it reasonable to use this population for drug study when it will not likely be able to benefit from the research? What will be the considerations regarding informed consent? Should local standards, which may be lax or nonexistent, be used? Should the researchers impose outside standards on the research? Are there obligations of the research team toward the medical community in the country where the testing occurs? (See reference 1.)

WORLD MEDICAL ASSOCIATION DECLARATION OF HELSINKI

Recommendations guiding physicians
in biomedical research involving human subjects

Adopted by the 18th World Medical Assembly
Helsinki, Finland, June 1964

and amended by the
29th World Medical Assembly, Tokyo, Japan, October 1975
35th World Medical Assembly, Venice, Italy, October 1983
and the
41st World Medical Assembly, Hong Kong, September 1989

© World Medical Association. Used with permission

INTRODUCTION

It is the mission of the physician to safeguard the health of the people. His or her knowledge and conscience are dedicated to the fulfillment of this mission.

The Declaration of Geneva of the World Medical Association binds the physician with the words, "The Health of my patient will be my first consideration," and the International Code of Medical Ethics declares that "A physician shall act only in the patient's interest when providing medical care which might have the effect of weakening the physical and mental condition of the patient."

The purpose of biomedical research involving human subjects must be to improve diagnostic, therapeutic and prophylactic procedures and the understanding of the aetiology and pathogenesis of disease.

In current medical practice most diagnostic, therapeutic or prophylactic procedures involve hazards. This applies especially to biomedical research.

Medical progress is based on research which ultimately must rest in part on experimentation involving human subjects.

In the field of biomedical research a fundamental distinction must be recognized between medical research in which the aim is essentially diagnostic or therapeutic for a patient, and medical research, the essential object of which is purely scientific and without implying direct diagnostic or therapeutic value to the person subjected to the research.

Special caution must be exercised in the conduct of research which may affect the environment, and the welfare of animals used for research must be respected.

Because it is essential that the results of laboratory experiments be applied to human beings to further scientific knowledge and to help suffering humanity, the World Medical Association has prepared the following recommendations as a guide to every physician in biomedical research involving human subjects. They should be kept under review in the future. It must be stressed that the standards as drafted are only a guide to physicians all over the world. Physicians are not relieved from criminal, civil and ethical responsibilities under the laws of their own countries.

I. BASIC PRINCIPLES

1. Biomedical research involving human subjects must conform to generally accepted scientific principles and should be based on adequately performed laboratory and animal experimentation and on a thorough knowledge of the scientific literature.

2. The design and performance of each experimental procedure involving human subjects should be clearly formulated in an experimental protocol which should be transmitted for consideration, comment and guidance to a specially appointed committee independent of the in-

vestigator and the sponsor provided that this independent committee is in conformity with the laws and regulations of the country in which the research experiment is performed.

3. Biomedical research involving human subjects should be conducted only by scientifically qualified persons and under the supervision of a clinically competent medical person. The responsibility for the human subject must always rest with a medically qualified person and never rest on the subject of the research, even though the subject has given his or her consent.

4. Biomedical research involving human subjects cannot legitimately be carried out unless the importance of the objective is in proportion to the inherent risk to the subject.

5. Every biomedical research project involving human subjects should be preceded by careful assessment of predictable risks in comparison with foreseeable benefits to the subject or to others. Concern for the interests of the subject must always prevail over the interests of science and society.

6. The right of the research subject to safeguard his or her integrity must always be respected. Every precaution should be taken to respect the privacy of the subject and to minimize the impact of the study on the subject's physical and mental integrity and on the personality of the subject.

7. Physicians should abstain from engaging in research projects involving human subjects unless they are satisfied that the hazards involved are believed to be predictable. Physicians should cease any investigation if the hazards are found to outweigh the potential benefits.

8. In publication of the results of his or her research, the physician is obliged to preserve the accuracy of the results. Reports of experimentation not in accordance with the principles laid down in this Declaration should not be accepted for publication.

9. In any research on human beings, each potential subject must be adequately informed of the aims, methods, anticipated benefits and potential hazards of the study and the discomfort it may entail. He or she should be informed that he or she is at liberty to abstain from participation in the study and that he or she is free to withdraw his or her consent to participation at any time. The physician should then obtain the subject's freely-given informed consent, preferably in writing.

10. When obtaining informed consent for the research project the physician should be particularly cautious if the subject is in a dependent relationship to him or her or may consent under duress. In that case the informed consent should be obtained by a physician who is not engaged in the investigation and who is completely independent of this official relationship.

11. In case of legal incompetence, informed consent should be obtained from the legal guardian in accordance with national legislation. Where physical or mental incapacity makes it impossible to obtain informed consent, or when the subject is a minor, permission from the responsible relative replaces that of the subject in accordance with national legislation.

    Whenever the minor child is in fact able to give a consent, the minor's consent must be obtained in addition to the consent of the minor's legal guardian.

12. The research protocol should always contain a statement of the ethical considerations involved and should indicate that the principles enunciated in the present Declaration are complied with.

II. MEDICAL RESEARCH COMBINED WITH PROFESSIONAL CARE (Clinical Research)

1. In the treatment of the sick person, the physician must be free to use a new diagnostic and therapeutic measure, if in his or her judgment it offers hope of saving life, reestablishing health or alleviating suffering.

2. The potential benefits, hazards and discomfort of a new method should be weighed against the advantages of the best current diagnostic and therapeutic methods.

3. In any medical study, every patient—including those of a control group, if any—should be assured of the best proven diagnostic and therapeutic method.

4. The refusal of the patient to participate in a study must never interfere with the physician-patient relationship.

5. If the physician considers it essential not to obtain informed consent, the specific reasons for the proposal should be stated in the experimental protocol of transmission to the independent committee (I, 2).

6. The physician can combine medical research with professional care, the objective being the acquisition of new medical knowledge, only to the extent that medical research is justified by its potential diagnostic or therapeutic value for the patient.

III. NON-THERAPEUTIC BIOMEDICAL RESEARCH INVOLVING HUMAN SUBJECTS (Non-Clinical Biomedical Research)

1. In the purely scientific application of medical research carried out on a human being, it is the duty of the physician to remain the protector of the life and health of that person on whom biomedical research is being carried out.

2. The subjects should be volunteers—either healthy persons or patients for whom the experimental design is not related to the patient's illness.
3. The investigator or the investigating team should discontinue the research if in his / her or their judgement it may, if continued, be harmful to the individual.
4. In research on man, the interest of science and society should never take precedence over considerations related to the wellbeing of the subject.

REFERENCES

The general reference used in preparation of this chapter was the *Code of Federal Regulations*, Title 45, Part 46, "Protection of Human Subjects." The publication *IRB: A Review of Human Subjects Research* also provides a wealth of practical and useful information for those interested in human research. Both are likely to be available at most institutional review board administrative offices.

1. **Barry, M., and M. Molyneux.** 1992. Ethical dilemmas in malaria drug and vaccine trials: a bioethical perspective. *J. Med. Ethics* **18**:189–192.
2. **Beecher, H. K.** 1966. Ethics and clinical research. *N. Engl. J. Med.* **274**:1354–1360.
3. **Begley, S., M. Hager, D. Glick, and J. Foote.** 1993. Cures from the womb, p. 49–51. *Newsweek*, February 22.
4. **Fulford, K. W. M., and K. Howse.** 1993. Ethics of research with psychiatric patients: principles, problems and the primary responsibilities of researchers. *J. Med. Ethics* **19**:85–91.
5. **Harth, S. C., R. R. Johnstone, and Y. H. Thong.** 1992. The psychological profile of parents who volunteer their children for clinical research: a controlled study. *J. Med. Ethics* **18**:86–93.
6. **Jones, J. H.** 1993. *Bad Blood, the Tuskegee Syphilis Experiment*. The Free Press, New York.
7. **Koren, G., D. B. Carmeli, Y. S. Carmeli, and R. Haslam.** 1993. Maturity of children to consent to medical research: the babysitter test. *J. Med. Ethics* **19**:142–147.
8. **Martin, D. K.** 1993. Abortion and fetal tissue transplantation, p. 1–3. *In IRB—A Review of Human Subjects Research*, Vol. 15. Hastings Center, Briarcliff Manor, NY.
9. **Ostini, R., G. Bammer, P. Dance, and R. E. Goodin.** 1993. The ethics of experimental heroin maintenance. *J. Med. Ethics* **19**:175–182.
10. **Riis, P.** 1993. Medical ethics in the European Community. *J. Med. Ethics* **19**:7–12.
11. **Woodward, K., M. Hayer, and D. Glick.** 1993. A search for limit, p. 52. *Newsweek*, February 22.

7 | *Conflict of Interest*

S. Gaylen Bradley

Introduction

Background

The professional life of a scientist involves choices on what problems to study, what methods to use, which literature to cite, how to collect and organize data, how to interpret data, and how results and interpretations are to be communicated and to whom. The scientist also faces choices on how much effort to devote to various research projects, to teaching, to public service, to professional service, to actual research, to identifying new problems, to interpreting data, to publicizing achievements, to managing and coordinating research, and to the search for funds to support the research enterprise. Numerous factors influence the decision on how scientists expend their effort. Some assignments come from the employer. Some decisions are influenced by the reward system, and some reflect individual personal qualities and background. The reward system for scientists is varied, including personal income, job security, prestige, funds for research, recognition by the public, power, and a personal sense of accomplishment (8). Most of the factors that influence the choices and behaviors of scientists are accepted as normal considerations in the decision-making process. The scientist is expected to weigh the merits of rewards that are given for conflicting goals and to arrive at decisions independent of personal interests. In reality, this is an internally incompatible admonition. At the present time, scientists are exhorted to contribute to the economic development of the nation. Proprietary interests call for restricted access to research directed to products of commercial value whereas the scientific tradition calls for openness,

161

free inquiry, and free exchange of ideas (11). A scientist is subject to a range of conflicting pressures that have different implications, including penalties for transgressions. These conflicting pressures may be categorized as conflicts of interest, conflicts of effort, and conflicts of conscience. There is a growing concern at this time in the public and in the scientific community about conflicts of interest.

Universities and their faculties enter into business relations with the private sector for a number of reasons, many of which are external to the university. The public and government sectors have seen commercialization of research as a means to create jobs that contribute to the gross domestic product and thereby generate tax revenues, to attract domestic and international investment, and to restore a favorable balance of trade by decreasing purchases of foreign goods and products and enhancing purchases of domestic goods and products. Universities and faculty scientists have seen partnerships with business as a new source of revenue for research, for university infrastructure, and for discretionary funds. The search for new sources of revenue has been viewed as particularly important during a period when federal funding of research and research training has been steadily decreasing (1).

Contractual arrangements between industry and a university or an academic investigator not only raise questions about specific conflicts of interest but also may change the overall intellectual climate in which academic researchers work. Universities and faculty members with a financial interest in commercial ventures may lose objectivity in making decisions. Academic science has extolled the virtue of a free exchange of ideas, sharing of data to accelerate scientific progress, and maintaining the quality of science by critical peer review at all stages of the scientific method. Individual scientists and university administrators may feel less inclined to discuss research at early stages if there is a perceived potential that economically valuable intellectual property may be generated. Secrecy is viewed by many as being contrary to academic science, a position taken by many socially conscious scientists as an argument against university-based research being funded by military agencies. There are divergent views about the impact of secrecy on the progress of science. There are those who feel that progress is retarded by the failure to have a free exchange of ideas and data. Others hold that the added resources for research with commercial value allow more workers to be recruited to the field, and that this accelerates achieving applied goals. This chapter describes a wide range of conflicts of interest (4).

Many science educators have expressed concern about the effects of industrially sponsored research on research training. One concern is that the attention devoted to scholarship with economic potential will lead research trainees to develop research strategies for short-term goals and modest extension of knowledge rather than formulating truly novel questions leading to major advances and changes in scientific thinking and problem solving. A related concern is that universities and faculty mentors will use research training to subsidize their commitments to industrial sponsors, and will give less attention to nurturing curiosity and innovation. The fear is that mentors will prize well-executed routine studies over creative exploration that goes beyond tried and true methodologies. In fact, students (by paying tuition and fees) and benefactors of the university may be unwittingly subsidizing commercial ventures.

Finally, there is a concern that this climate of secrecy and economic competition is contributing to a loss of public confidence in the integrity of science and scientists, if not to an actual deterioration in the quality of science. There is, however, no established correlation between recent incidents of scientific falsification, fabrication, or plagiarism and economic conflict of interest. In fact, many of the additional procedures demanded in research associated with industry (for example, careful record keeping, and review of results by a colleague) tend to prevent falsification and fabrication of data. Nevertheless, the perception that scientists today are less rigorous and self-critical is widely held by the public, news media, legislators, and even the scientific community itself (14).

Definitions

Conflict of interest is a legal term which encompasses a wide spectrum of behaviors or actions involving personal gain or financial interest. The definition of conflict of interest (including the scope of persons subject to the provisions in a code or set of rules and regulations) varies according to state and federal statutes, case law, contracts of employment, professional standards of conduct, and agreements between affected parties or corporations or both. A conflict of interest exists when an individual exploits his or her position for personal gain or for the profit of a member of his or her immediate family or household. The identification of members of the immediate family and household is in a state of flux, but these individuals include the spouse and minor children living at home. Case law is evolving with respect to dependent parents and "significant other" persons. Another critical component of conflict of interest pertains to the undue use of a position or exercise of power to influence a decision for personal gain. Many conflict of interest codes also prohibit activities that create an appearance of a conflict of interest. Full disclosure may be the only means to combat perceptions of undue influence. Conflict of interest is distinctly different from conflict of effort and conflict of conscience and these will be discussed in detail later. An individual may, however, become entangled in more than one of these conflicts as a result of participation in a single activity. Conflict of interest is also distinctly different from bias in research, which is the inability or unwillingness to consider alternative approaches or interpretations on their own merits. Scientists sometimes develop strong preferences for particular research techniques, or become deeply vested in a particular working model to the exclusion of alternative explanations. The origin of these prejudices may be subconscious, or at least unrecognized, reflecting past training, cultural background, experience, or group dynamics (7).

Legislative bodies, governing boards, and the public have tended to define and specify penalties for conflict of interest in science by a single code. There is little recognition of a hierarchy of injury to the public well-being. Clearly, however, the public is harmed to a far greater extent when a conflict of interest is allowed to influence a clinical decision to market a drug for human use than when a conflict of interest is allowed to influence the decision to purchase an item of laboratory equipment from a particular vendor or to hire a relative to work in the laboratory of a scientist.

The changing climate
The federal government has taken a number of actions that encourage universities to enter into agreements with the private sector, thereby creating circumstances that ensnare faculty in potential or real conflicts of interest. The 1980 Bayh–Dole Act (Patent and Trademark Laws Amendment, Public Law 96-517) allows a federal contractor to take ownership of the property rights for inventions created in the pursuit of a grant or contract. The Bayh-Dole Act specifies that income from the exploitation of these intellectual properties must be shared with

the inventor and the remainder used for scientific research or educational purposes (10). The Federal Technology Transfer Act of 1986 extended the incentives for collaboration with industry to technology developed in a government laboratory. This act allows government laboratories to enter into cooperative research and economic development agreements (CRADAs) with other governmental agencies and with nongovernmental profit and nonprofit organizations. Income from inventions developed under a CRADA are shared with the government inventor, and the remainder is to be used by the participating company for technology transfer (9).

The biomedical research enterprise expanded dramatically during the mid-1950s to mid-1970s. Since the 1970s, funding from federal agencies such as the National Institutes of Health has increased only modestly, and has remained at the same level, in terms of constant dollars, for the past 5 to 10 years (12). During the past decade, health care costs and other demands on state and federal funds have increased sharply, forcing scientists and research administrators to look for alternative sources of funding. Concurrently, biotechnology has emerged as a significant economic force, with the potential to contribute substantially to the gross domestic product and to the international balance of trade. Scientists have been encouraged by government and academic employers to enter into university–industry ventures and to be entrepreneurs in commercializing new technologies. University employers have seen technology transfer as a new source of revenue to replace decreasing support from state and federal agencies. At the local level, many communities have developed economic plans in which research parks are the means to provide jobs, tax revenues, and economic vitality for their regions.

Conflict of Interest

Orientation

Basic research workers have a tradition of free inquiry and free exchange of ideas, united in a shared purpose to create knowledge, to critique existing knowledge, and to disseminate knowledge. The image of the eccentric scientist lacking worldly aspirations and living in a cloistered ivory tower is giving way to that of a greedy entrepreneur who is insensitive to the public good. Science and science administrators have promised, and the public has come to expect, products of research and technology that improve the quality of life. The public has called upon scientists to discover means to prevent or cure cancer, heart disease, mental illness, and AIDS and lavishes great rewards upon those who appear to achieve these goals. It is a small wonder then that many scientists have lost their ingenuousness and fallen afoul of conflicts of interest (5).

Equity interests
Members of the academic scientific community receive conflicting admonitions from government, employers, and the public. Scientists are urged to accelerate the transfer of basic science knowledge into application and commercialization. The public has expressed concern that science is not sufficiently responsive to public need and that the lag from laboratory discovery to application is too long. National, state, and local governments, and business communities, have turned to research as the means to maintain economic competitiveness. Scientists quickly learn that most of their research discoveries with potential for commercialization require substantial development before established industry is willing to invest in university-generated intellectual property. Scientists who are convinced of the market potential of their inventions soon find that the patent process and product development are expensive and time-consuming. In addition, most scientists lack experience in writing a business plan and in securing venture capital. Quite often, the scientist will enter into an entrepreneurial corporation as an equity owner. Scientists inevitably feel that they are the most qualified to lead the technical development of the invention. It is at this stage that concerns about conflict of interest arise. In general, public institutions restrict the circumstances under which scientist–entrepreneurs may receive grants or contracts through their universities from a corporation in which they are in management positions or equity owners or both. Private institutions usually have fewer restrictions on faculty entrepreneurship than do public institutions. It is imperative that faculty entrepreneurs disclose possible conflict-of-interest situations to their administrations. Failure to do so, or intentionally withholding information about potential conflict of interest situations constitutes a violation of the rules and procedures of most universities (2).

Compensation
Academic scientists are employed by their institutions to teach, to conduct research, and to render service to the institution, surrounding

community, and the profession itself. The relative effort in each activity varies according to the mission of the institution and according to strategies to utilize effectively the talents of the faculty. Faculty members who are actively engaged in research have the opportunity to present their results to colleagues, including those who are employed by for-profit corporations. In general, universities encourage faculty members to present seminars and lectures at other research centers, and condone payment of speakers fees and full reimbursement of travel expenses. Scientists whose research bears upon commercial application of a product may be invited to conferences targeting groups that influence purchasing decisions. A scientist studying the mechanism of action of an antibiotic may be invited to participate in a conference, sponsored by the pharmaceutical company distributing the antibiotic, targeted to physicians who will prescribe the drug. The scientist may be paid a generous speaker's fee or honorarium and provided luxury travel and lodging accommodations. There is a broad spectrum of speaker's fees, honoraria, and travel accommodations, some of which have attracted the attention of the Internal Revenue Service as well as the public. Honoraria and speaker's fees above a modest level are increasingly scrutinized by employers, especially academic administrators.

Consultantships are a formal agreement between a scientist and a corporation other than his or her primary employer, and usually with a for-profit company. Consultants have played critical roles in technology transfer, and academic scientists gain insights into the needs of industry for personnel and basic research. In general, consultantships have been beneficial to all parties: industry, the university, and the individual scientist. Consultantship arrangements are usually reviewed and subject to approval by one's employer; however, there are a number of valid concerns associated with them. A scientist–consultant must not transmit to a private business information, records, or materials generated as a result of research sponsored by benevolent foundations or governmental agencies unless the same information, records, or materials are made readily available to the scientific community in general. This guideline does not preclude appropriate contractual arrangements among the research sponsor, the research institution, and a private firm, particularly in the context of a licensing agreement (15). A consultantship should be based upon the collective knowledge and experience of the scientist and not constitute a means to gain access to privileged or confidential information available to the scientist by virtue of his / her employment or professional activities on advisory boards. A scientist–consultant must assiduously avoid the appearance of a conflict of interest whenever the employer is negotiating a contract with the private organization with which the scientist is a paid consultant. Scientist–consultants have the responsibility to disclose to their employers any agreements to perform consulting services. Moreover, they should not participate as evaluators of grant or contract proposals submitted by companies for whom they serve as consultants (3).

Gifts and gratuities
Scientists have considerable influence on procurement decisions, including equipment and services. Vendors use a number of inducements to convince scientists and purchasing agents of the merits of their products or customer services. Exhibitors at national professional meetings hold breakfasts and receptions, and give out carrying cases and a variety of mementos to establish product recognition in the minds of scientists. These modest gifts and gratuities have become routine, accepted, and expected. Vendors also give books and videotapes, and host formal lunches and dinners. At some point, meals and entertainment cross from modest mementos to serious inducements. Currently, frequent flyer credits are a widely used inducement and various employers have taken different positions regarding this practice. There is no doubt that some scientists select an airline carrier according to accumulation of frequent flyer credits rather than cost or convenience. When this occurs, the scientist has allowed a personal interest to conflict with the interests of the employer (19).

There is no sharp boundary between gifts and compensation. Is the biomedical scientist who is fully reimbursed to attend a conference receiving compensation, a gift, or gratuity? Scientific leaders are sometimes invited to attend a conference, not to give a formal lecture but to lend prestige and credibility to the program. Bench scientists may be invited to clinical conferences to lend the aura of solid scientific underpinning even though the scientists may have no direct experience with the drug or clinical trial. Local scientists may be invited to a conference to build community goodwill or to fill the audience or both. There are no universally applicable guidelines to delineate the boundary between professional courtesy and a personal perquisite that has fiscal implications and the potential to influence a decision.

Clearly America's free economy relies heavily upon advertising, promotion, and inducements to influence purchasing choices. Scientists are confronted with the dichotomy that what is proper as an inducement to purchase a home television is usually not proper as an inducement to influence selection of a television monitor at work.

Multiple pay for one job

As relationships for the conduct of research become more complex, several sources of financial support are used to pay for research, especially that having potential commercial value. A university-based scientist, paid primarily by institutional funds, may conduct research on a project supported by a federal agency such as the National Institutes of Health. In addition, the scientist may hold a paid leadership position in a venture company which has a contract with the university supporting research in the same laboratory for the same or closely related study. It may not be clear whether or not the scientist is being paid by his/her employer and by a for-profit corporation for technical guidance of the same research. Most universities insist on documentation that employees are not being paid twice for the same job assignment. This usually involves documentation of the management role of the scientist in the leadership of the venture company.

Nepotism

Most state and federal agencies are subject to statutes or have rules that preclude a scientist from hiring or supervising an immediate member of his/her family or of the same household. These statutes are, in part, rooted in strategies to ensure fair access to employment opportunities. One of the most frequent nepotism practices is hiring high school or college-age progeny by an investigator, particularly for part-time and summer work. This practice is clearly contrary to equal access to employment opportunities and career development for underrepresented groups. In addition, selection of immediate members of the family for employment constitutes use of a position of authority for personal gain. Similarly, exercise of an investigator's authority to hire a member of his/her family has multiple implications for equal employment opportunity and personal financial benefit. The boundaries of propriety are not always well delineated. A few organizations prohibit members of the same family from working in the same department, even though neither party has direct authority over the other's selection, promotion, or salary. With a growing number of two-career families, this limits the ability to recruit highly competent professionals to some institutions. A few institutions, on the other hand, have made concerted efforts to recruit two-career families. There are risks, however. The careers of the two individuals may not advance in parallel and a two-career couple may make personal decisions about their relationship that cause tensions in the workplace. The organizational distance between members of a family or household in the workplace is not well defined. Is a faculty member permitted to select a member of the household of a departmental chair, dean, or vice president for a position in the faculty member's laboratory? The definition of member of the immediate family or household has occasionally been broadened to encompass individuals with a significant personal relationship but who are not "blood relatives" or married. Nepotism regulations will undoubtedly remain in a state of flux as the goals of equal access to employment and career opportunities conflict with the career aspirations of two-career families. The American Association of University Professors has called for the discontinuation of policies and practices that proscribe the opportunities for the members of an immediate family from serving as professional colleagues (16).

Scientific conflict of interest

A successful scientist is afforded the opportunity to participate in the decisionmaking process that influences the allocation of resources. The peer review system, which is considered one of the essential safeguards for the quality of science, can be abused to serve a personal interest. Members of editorial boards have occasionally been accused of delaying publication of the results of a competitor in order to gain priority and recognition that strengthens applications for funding from granting agencies. Members of editorial boards have also been accused of being uncritical of manuscripts presenting results favoring a method or product in which the reviewer has a personal interest. Authors sometimes feel that reviewers have been unduly critical of manuscripts that describe in a favorable light products competing with one in which the reviewer has a personal interest. There is growing concern within the scientific community about the prudence of allowing employees of commercial firms to review manuscripts evaluating methods or products having economic value or potential. Some journals which publish articles related to commercial methods or products are asking both authors and reviewers to disclose their financial interests. Many scientists have felt that these requirements have impuned their integrity, and in most instances that their financial interests are proportionally so modest that they cannot be considered a "substantial personal interest." Nevertheless, concern about the perception of conflict of interest is growing, especially in biomedical fields, and demands for financial disclosure by scientists are apt to increase (8).

Most grant review panels and advisory boards have established conflict of interest guidelines. The National Institutes of Health asks individuals evaluating grant or contract proposals and applications to avoid reviewing submissions from organizations in which they (1) have a financial interest, (2) are directors, officers, consultants, or employees, or (3) are prospective employees or shareholders. The admonition extends to holdings of spouses and minor children, and even to circumstances in which there is an apparent conflict of interest. Members of National Institutes of Health study sections are not allowed to review applications from their own institutions or those of a former student, professional collaborator, close personal friend, or colleague with whom the evaluator has long-standing or personal differences. If the excluded category is too large, the most knowledgeable reviewers are not allowed to participate in the decisionmaking process. The risk of inept evaluation by less informed reviewers must be weighed against the adverse effects of a perceived conflict of interest. Unsuccessful applicants for research grants occasionally feel that a competitor on a study section has been unduly critical in order to gain an edge in recognition and future funding. The National Institutes of Health has developed an appeals process to handle complaints of alleged unfair review of grant applications.

Scientists are increasingly being called upon to serve as experts for executive, legislative, and judicial deliberations. In addition, they have sought opportunities to testify before legislative committees that appropriate funds for research and higher education. Legislators, in turn, have come to view scientists as lobbyists or trade union representatives, advocating self-interest rather than public interests. The scientific community itself is divided over the propriety of direct appeals to fund scientific projects outside of the peer review system by congressionally earmarked or "pork barrel" appropriations. Scientists engaged in expert testimony before the courts have encountered an adversial culture unlike scholarly debate. Sometimes they are unwilling expert witnesses who have been subpoenaed to present evidence and research results (13). Scientists who willingly serve as expert witnesses for pay have been accused of conflicts of interest and even of giving misleading information. Advisory boards of executive agencies have increasingly insisted on disclosure of past and present financial interests and have excluded persons with financial interests in a product or the company that manufactures it. The threshold for determining a perceived conflict of interest varies, and sometimes is set so low that it leads to the exclusion of scientists whose financial interests have been limited to speaker's fees and associated reimbursement of expenses. The assessment of the risk of advice from a less knowledgeable panel against the adverse effects of perceived conflict of interest is often made in the context of the political sensitivity of the issue rather than the needs of the decisionmaking process (20).

Academic conflict of interest

Academic scientists have specific responsibilities to protect academic freedom, to disseminate knowledge, to maintain academic standards, to critique the current state of knowledge, to synthesize existing knowledge, and to apply knowledge to solve basic and applied problems. Faculty members are increasingly called upon to link the educational process to fund-raising and revenue-generating enterprises. Research faculty members are sometimes encouraged to market their expertise by organizing and presenting profitable workshops, particularly for business firms, under the auspices of the university. In other instances, faculty members have independently developed for-profit short courses and used the net earnings as a source of personal income. At some point these entrepreneurial activities, which are not restricted to academic scientists, have the potential to constitute a conflict of interest in which the faculty members utilize the reputation and even the resources of their employer for personal gain. In addition, the time and energy devoted to these activities may lead to a conflict of effort.

Corporations and wealthy individuals may want to use their resources to influence the direction of academic programs. An agribusiness corporation may want to endow a chair in human nutrition, and a grateful patient may want to endow a chair in transplantation biology. Universities have developed sophisticated infrastructures to enhance these sources of support, and may give prizes to alumni and business leaders, not totally without consideration that the grateful recipients might generously support the university in the future. Gifts that are consistent with the mission of the university are aggressively sought. Agreements that proffer undue personal benefit to the donor, the university, or an employee of the university may, however, constitute a conflict of interest.

Academic degrees have economic value, and progress toward completion of a degree can become an issue in a conflict of interest. In an earlier section, an example was given in which a faculty advisor extended the course of study of a student to benefit a corporate sponsor. Companies sometimes use opportunities to obtain advanced degrees as an employee benefit and perquisite to stabilize staff retention. Companies usually place limits on the time that they will pay for educational leaves or release from work time. The duration of educational leaves is usually inadequate for the average student to complete the degree program in the standard depth for other students. The student and the student's supervisor in the company sponsoring the educational leave may put pressure on the advisor to make exceptions and to waive requirements. These requests may be linked to hints of benefits to the advisor and institution once the employee graduates and returns to his or her regular or more influential position in the company.

Institutional conflict of interest

Institutions acquire financial interests in the private sector through earnings on intellectual property, exclusive contracts with industry, and equity ownership in a for-profit company. In general, the interests of scientist–inventors and their employing institutions are congruent with respect to earnings on intellectual property. When the scientist and the institution share in revenues based upon a predetermined rate, the more successful the product, the better each fares. There are several areas in which the scientist and the institution may have conflicting interests. The scientist may seek a generous consulting arrangement as part of a licensing agreement. The institution may have limitations on this type of consulting arrangement, or may seek other concessions from the company seeking a license at the expense of the scientist's self-interest. Similarly, scientists may seek research and development funds for their laboratories as a part of licensing agreements. This entails assigning rights of first refusal to the licensing company, a commitment about which the scientist and the employing institution may have divergent views. In addition, the institution may have restrictions on this type of grant or contract, particularly if it involves assessment of the efficacy of the invention or product. Moreover, the institution and the licensing company may feel that the invention will be developed more rapidly and to a greater extent without the parallel participation of the inventor (6).

Institutions have been entering into exclusive contracts with industry to give preferential access to research results to a company. The company usually awards the institution a large multiyear umbrella award. Invention disclosures are called to the attention of the sponsoring company, and technology transfer officers of the university may encourage scientists to work in areas of interest to the company. Several conflicts have arisen from these blanket agreements between a company and an institution. Any one company, regardless of its size, has a reasonably well-defined scope. Scientists whose inventions lie outside the interest of the company may not receive adequate assistance from their employing institution in patenting and licensing efforts. There is a potential conflict between scientists whose work is supported by other commercial firms and the institution, which is striving to fulfill its contract to the company with an exclusive agreement. There is also growing concern that funds from government agencies and from tax-exempt foundations are being used to subsidize preferentially the research and development of for-profit companies, many of which are foreign owned.

Universities too are being offered equity interest in entrepreneurial ventures involving faculty members. A research institution that accepts an equity position in a start-up company is likely to offer encouragement to the scientist entrepreneur at critical times. In addition, the investors are not depleted of cash necessary for successful development and marketing of the product, and the ultimate return to the university has the potential to exceed income from royalties and licensing fees. University administrators, in such circumstances, find themselves called upon to make decisions in which the interests of the venture corporation and those of the university faculty may not be identical. University administrators may become unduly interested in the economic success of the venture company, even at the expense of educational responsibilities of the university. There is also a question of whether or not an institution that holds equity in a commercial venture will allow that financial interest to influence staffing decisions or other allocations of resources. When a position becomes vacant, will the employer preferentially seek candidates who will contribute to the development of the product in which the employer has an interest? When decisions on the allocation of limited resources for the purchase of equipment are made, will research administrators favor those units working on proprietary projects in which the employer has an interest?

Universities are under increasing pressure to take equity in start-up companies based upon the intellectual property of one of their own faculty. The institution may provide release time for the faculty member, technical assistance for the project, and access to equipment and other research infrastructure in return for substantial ownership in the company. Proponents of equity ownership by institutions emphasize that this is an inexpensive investment with the potential for enormous economic returns. Opponents of equity ownership by institutions argue that institutional resources are diverted to the personal benefit of one or two scientists and the investors in the venture capital deal. The equity-owning institution has an exceptional interest in the success of the venture, and may use its research and public relations resources to promote a venture without adequate safeguards on fiduciary responsibility or critical scientific peer review. It is clear that equity ownership of companies based upon the research of the scientists of an institution is coming under increased public scrutiny, legal challenges from other members of the institution, and restrictive regulations from federal funding agencies (18).

Institutional prerogatives
Universities have a strong sense of self-preservation or self-protection when confronted with issues that are likely to have a major adverse effect on the institution. They may be reluctant to cancel lucrative contracts when a faculty member is found to have a serious conflict of interest. The reputation of leading research universities is based upon extramural support and achievements that attract positive public attention, such as patents, prizes received by faculty, and scientific breakthroughs of general interest. Universities are thus threatened in two ways by scientific misconduct: the potential loss of grant funds and the loss of prestige. In addition, an investigation of scientific mis-

conduct is expensive. As a result, universities are not typically eager to invite complaints of scientific misconduct or conflict of interest.

The bureaucrats within the university are certainly reluctant to be drawn into proceedings pertaining to scientific misconduct or conflict of interest. Administrators are insecure about their mastery of the process, are fearful of political repercussions within the institution when a distinguished scientist is the subject of a complaint, and are anxious about criticism from news media, which frequently focuses on individuals rather than issues. Colleagues within the university are also reluctant to become involved in deliberations about conflict of interest or scientific misconduct because it is perceived as taking sides with the complainant or the alleged perpetrator. Scientists are also aware of the potential financial damage to their institution, and the negative effect on the institution's image, and feel some need to protect their employer and to attenuate adverse effects of the allegation.

Taken as a whole, universities not only have failed to take the lead in addressing scientific misconduct and conflict of interest, but have been perceived by the news media and some legislators as inept and even recalcitrant in assuming responsibility for the behavior of the members of their community. Universities are particularly concerned about the increasing administrative responsibilities assigned to them by state and federal governments, because many of these requirements are perceived as placing university administrators at odds with the attitudes and aspirations of their own scientists. There is little doubt, however, that the public and legislators will increasingly insist that universities accept responsibility for monitoring the integrity of the science carried out by their employees and trainees, and for the personal interests of employees that may affect the independence of decisionmaking. Judgments on these complex issues are best vested in those who understand the standards of the discipline and the particular environment in which the conduct being examined occurs.

Conflict of Effort

Conflict of effort is distinctly different from conflict of interest, although the same set of external circumstances may precipitate both dilemmas. A conflict of effort arises when demands made by parties other than the primary employer interfere with the performance of the employee's assigned duties in teaching, research, and service. In general, scientists are expected to notify their employer of outside responsibilities, to seek permission in advance in most instances, and to report annually on outside professional activities, whether paid or not. Scientists with successful research programs are asked to present seminars and lectures at other institutions, at conferences, and at meetings. They are also asked to serve on editorial boards, research advisory panels, and policy advisory boards. They may be asked to teach in short courses and to offer methods workshops for peers or professionals in related fields. The university employer encourages some participation in these activities and uses them as criteria in evaluation for promotion, salary increases, and tenure decisions. Good things can be carried to excess, however, and virtually every research-intense university has a number of faculty spending an unacceptable amount of time away from campus. A conflict of effort is serious when the scientist is not available for scheduled classes, for student advising, for guidance of research trainees, for oversight of research projects and resource accountability, and for assigned administrative and service duties. Most universities allow 20% of a faculty member's effort or one day per week for consultation and outside professional activity. Some entrepreneurial faculty members try to define this limitation only in terms of paid consultantships and income-generating outside professional activity, and do not report professional service or speaking engagements that are unpaid or only reimbursed for expenses. This is not the intent of policies on outside professional activities, which are more concerned about faculty effort than faculty compensation. There are those who believe that it is the neglect of, or inattention to, assigned duties at the employing institution that has allowed charges of scientific misconduct to come to public attention (2).

To avoid a conflict of effort, a scientist ought to review assigned duties with his/her supervisor and discuss the effort involved and the value to the department, institution, or profession. In general, the immediate supervisor (for example, a department chair) is responsible for orchestrating the resources of the unit and for the appropriate deployment of personnel. The immediate supervisor, however, is not usually the person with primary responsibility for making decisions on conflict of interest, although he or she should have a role in alerting the administrator responsible for managing conflict of interest of a potential problem. Immediate supervisors usually lack the legal knowledge to interpret conflict of interest regulations.

Some of the more difficult conflicts of effort also involve conflict of interest. Scientists who establish for-profit companies may experience increasing demands on their time that interfere with their ability to fulfill assigned duties. What makes these decisions difficult is that the faculty members may be on site, but their effort may be directed to the interests of the private companies rather than toward the needs of the primary employer. In addition, the faculty member may meet scheduled assignments but arrive inadequately prepared. The faculty member may be inattentive to his/her advisory roles for students, staff, and research trainees. The immediate supervisor has the responsibility to counsel the faculty member about these concerns. After mutual agreement, if possible, on the extent of the problem, a date for a follow-up review should be set. If the faculty member and the immediate supervisor cannot reach a mutual accord, the matter may have to be considered by a grievance or disciplinary process.

Most conflicts of effort arise from the enthusiastic aspirations of scientists to gain acceptance from their peers and to achieve national and international stature as an investigator rather than from being secondary to conflicts of interest. Universities in particular send mixed messages to young faculty, placing a premium on professional recognition. Faculty members usually respond well to discussion of the expected balance of effort among teaching, research, and service. It is too much to expect young scientists to find the proper balance without role models, mentors, and guidance.

Conflict of Conscience

A third category of conflict, distinct from conflicts of interest or effort, has been recognized as conflict of conscience. A conflict of conscience does not involve financial reward or personal gain, and in all likelihood does not interfere with effort in assigned areas of teaching, research, and service, although it may affect performance in one or more of these areas. A conflict of conscience arises when the convictions of an individual override other considerations in reaching a decision. A scientist who abhors abortion and use of fetal tissue may be unable to act dispassionately on any manuscript or grant application that utilizes fetal tissue. A scientist who opposes all research using laboratory animals may be unable to find merit in any study or report that is based upon laboratory animals. These very personal views may not be known to colleagues at the same institution or elsewhere. Conflicts of conscience are not invariably viewed in a negative light. Scientists have occasionally refused to work on projects believed to be immoral applications of science, for example, development of infectious agents for biological warfare, or testing toxicity of drugs in uninformed human subjects such as mental patients, other institutionalized or incarcerated persons, or military personnel. To date, there is no agreement on whether or how to assess conflicts of conscience (17). As with other biases in reviewing manuscripts and grant applications, it is likely that responsible leadership would try to identify and correct any behavior that showed a pattern markedly at variance with other members of the deliberative process. Attempts to resolve conflicts of conscience as they relate to academic matters are apt to raise issues of abridgment of academic freedom. In the academic health science center, delivery of patient care is increasingly confronted with changing patterns of medical ethics with respect to premature births, resuscitation, life support systems, pain control, and suicide. Medical ethics committees have been formed in academic health care centers and other large health care systems, but parallel academic committees or procedures to deal with scientific conflicts of conscience are very rare. Public interest groups are, however, increasingly insistent on the right to sit on institutional bodies that review laboratory animal use, human subjects committees, environmental and occupational health and safety committees, and medical ethics committees.

Conclusion

Conflict of interest is an umbrella term for a wide range of behaviors and circumstances. At some level, it involves use of position or authority for personal gain. Although most attention has been directed toward personal financial gain by individuals, universities and other corporations may engage in practices that create a conflict of interest between the organization and individuals, most often its own employees, or with other corporations. Conflict of interest is distinctly different from conflict of effort and conflict of conscience. Conflict of effort pertains to allocation of time on behalf of the primary employer. Although conflict of effort may arise from the same activity that creates a conflict of interest, more often, a conflict of effort arises from diversion of the commitment of an individual by requests to engage in public service and outside professional activities. At some point, service on advisory boards, governing boards of professional and public organizations, and editorial boards, and participation in seminars, symposia, conferences, and workshops will impair the ability of individuals to meet their responsibilities to their employer, subordinates, trainees, and colleagues.

Some financial conflicts of interest are obvious. Others are not necessarily obvious and are defined by statutes. Still others are gauged by professional standards that vary with time or across disciplines. Various arbitrary thresholds have been established in statutes, institutional guidelines, and federal regulations that define the level of financial interest that creates a conflict of interest. Some laws may forbid activities or entering into contracts that create a conflict of interest; for example, an employee of a state agency may not receive more that $10,000 in compensation from an outside contractor doing business with that state agency. Most often, the individual is required to disclose a financial interest that may be perceived as creating a conflict of interest. Increasingly, a symposium speaker receiving a consulting fee from a pharmaceutical company is required to disclose that arrangement to the organizers and audience as a prerequisite to participation in a conference addressing the merits of the company's commercial products.

Scientific conflict of interest involves the use of position to influence decisions on publication of manuscripts, funding of grant applications, and formulation of regulations on the use or commercialization of a product. There is no general agreement on the circumstances that can create a scientific conflict of interest. Should a scientist employed by a pharmaceutical company be appointed to the editorial board of a journal that publishes articles on the efficacy of therapeutic agents? Should a scientist review the grant application of a collaborator or a competitor? Clearly, the definition of scientific conflict of interest cannot be made so broad as to exclude most individuals knowledgeable in the field from the evaluation process.

Institutional conflict of interest is less well defined than individual conflict of interest. An institutional conflict of interest arises when the interests of a university diverge from those of its faculty and staff. Most notable of these is an exclusive contract between a university and a corporation, giving the corporation preferential access to research results. Universities are increasingly becoming co-owners of companies established to commercialize the results of faculty research. There is a growing concern in some sectors that this commitment to economic development is leading universities away from their traditional roles as educational and scholarly sanctuaries.

Case Studies

7.1   A scientist is a consultant for a for-profit firm that manufactures a particular pesticide. The scientist is an internationally renowned authority on the toxicology of this pesticide. He is asked to serve on a federal advisory panel that is to address the need to regulate use and sale of this pesticide. The scientist seeks your advice. What do you tell your colleague?

7.2   An internationally renowned biomedical scientist is an authority in her field. She serves on a National Institutes of Health study section (10 days per year), a state advisory panel (10 days per year), a federal advisory panel (10 days per year), and an international advisory panel (10 days per year) and gives about one seminar a month at research universities across the country. What conflict of interest or conflict of effort considerations, if any, apply to this scenario?

7.3   Two scientists are recruited to a research university. After several years of professional association, they develop a romantic relationship that leads to marriage. Subsequently, one of the pair becomes the supervisor of the unit. What conflict of interest considerations, if any, apply to this scenario? What options are available to this two-career family?

7.4   A biomedical investigator is funded by a research grant from the National Science Foundation. The investigator has a college-age child who is majoring in a science discipline. The investigator proposes to employ her dependent for the summer to work on the project. The experience will be valuable for the college student, and the investigator will be assured of a reliable summer worker. What conflict of interest considerations, if any, apply to this scenario?

7.5   Dr. Cox at Research University is a renowned clinical pharmacologist. He has a large, productive research program in experimental therapeutics, sponsored by federal grants and industrial contracts. His reputation is such that his participation in a conference attracts news media attention and a large attendance. Big Company engages Dr. Cox for a series of lectures at conferences designed to promote Big Co.'s new therapeutic agent. Dr. Cox is paid a speaker's fee of $25,000 and all expenses for each presentation. Dr. Cox is free to select his topic and the contents of his presentation. Dr. Cox makes five to six appearances per year at Big Co.'s conferences. Comment on potential conflicts associated with the lecture series.

7.6 Dr. Oak is on the grants review panel of a major biomedical foundation. Dr. Oak's former student, Dr. Pine, now an associate professor at State University, submits a grant application which is sent to Dr. Oak to review. Dr. Oak has had little contact with Dr. Pine for the past five years, since Dr. Pine completed her postdoctoral training at a nearby university and moved to State University, located on the opposite corner of the country. Dr. Pine's research has taken significantly different directions than that of her former adviser, but Dr. Oak is well qualified to review the grant. Should Dr. Oak return the grant application to the foundation, review the application but note that he was Dr. Pine's advisor, or review the application with no comment that he was her advisor?

7.7 Dr. Knight at Research University has developed a genetically engineered vaccine. The work was supported by federal grants, and much of the research was carried out by graduate teaching assistants as part of their degree requirements. Research University negotiates a contract with Large Company to develop and market the vaccine. The contract pays 20% of Dr. Knight's salary for a commensurate part of Dr. Knight's effort. Dr. Knight owns 3% of Large Co.'s stock, is on the board of directors of Large Co., and is a paid consultant to the research director of Large Co. Members of the board of directors receive a modest $50 per day and all expenses for participating in the two-day board meetings held quarterly. You are asked to review and comment on Dr. Knight's disclosure report to her institution.

7.8 Dr. Elman at Research University has a federally funded project on synthesis and characterization of materials used to fabricate prosthetic devices. Major Company employs Dr. Elman as a consultant on the characteristics of its biomaterials, some of which are being marketed and some of which are in the development stage. Dr. Elman signs an agreement that she will not disclose confidential, proprietary information that she obtains from Major Co. Dr. Elman learns, as a consultant, that Major Co. plans to market a biomaterial that she has discovered in her research to have adverse properties. She notifies Major Co. of her findings during a consulting visit. Major Co. asks her to delay reporting these results in her progress report to her federal funding agency. Is this an appropriate request?

7.9 Research University negotiates a research and development contract with Important Company. Important Co. adds some of its own financial resources to the contract to select a postdoctoral research worker, who would officially be an employee of Research University. Important Co. and Research University are several hundred miles apart, and there is no other internship, practicum, or cooperative agreement between them. Research University delegates to Important Co. all oversight for supervision, evaluation, and compliance to occupational health and safety standards. Important Co. recruits an international scholar, who is paid a standard stipend but receives no health insurance or other benefits from either Important Co. or Research University. What are the potential conflicts involved?

7.10 Professor Maple at Research University is active in applied research and graduate training. He is funded primarily by research and development contracts from federal agencies. The project officer for one of the federal agencies, Mr. Rose, has a bachelor's degree and requires a master's degree for career advancement. Mr. Rose applies for, and is admitted to, the graduate program at Research University in which Professor Maple is a faculty member. Professor Maple works out an easy course of study for Mr. Rose, who quickly completes the required courses. Professor Maple then provides Mr. Rose with progress reports to be used as the bases for his master's thesis. Mr. Rose is grateful for the opportunity and is a strong advocate for renewal of Professor Maple's contract with the federal agency. Is this a conflict of interest? What other types of conflict may be involved?

7.11 Dr. White at Research University is organizing an international conference. Significant Company has an outstanding meeting facility which would be ideal for the conference. Dr. White asks the management of Significant Co. if they would make their meeting facility available. The management of Significant Co. indicates that they will co-sponsor the international conference, and asks that their research director, Dr. Jones, be given a prominent role in the program. Significant

Co. will also provide each conference participant with samples of its products, none of which is directly related to the topic of the conference. In addition, Significant Co. offers to host a reception and banquet for the participants at no cost. The president of Significant Co., however, would make a brief after-dinner speech, reviewing the corporate history of Significant Co. Should Dr. White agree to these arrangements? What concerns might conference participants have about them?

7.12 Dr. Allan at Research University has invented a biomedical instrument to monitor and record data on injured subjects being transported in an emergency vehicle to a hospital. Dr. Allan meets Mr. Ball, who is a venture capitalist. Mr. Ball is interested in Dr. Allan's invention and forms a company to develop and market the invention. Dr. Allan is given stock in the new company, and is assigned responsibility to monitor technical development of the invention. The new company enters into a contract with Research University to develop Dr. Allan's invention. Dr. Allan assigns his master's student, who is a graduate teaching assistant, to work on the project. Mr. Ball objects to the inclusion of some of the student's results in the master's thesis, and Dr. Allan removes the section in question. The student is required by Dr. Allan to complete additional work to meet degree requirements. Is this fair to the student? What types of conflict might come into play?

7.13 Dr. Victor at Research University has discovered and developed a new genetically engineered product of great potential value. A biotechnology company has been formed to produce and market the product. Administrators at Research University, being aware of the progress of the venture, buy considerable stock in the company. Research University also allocates additional space and personnel to Dr. Victor for her research on the product. The product is economically successful and Dr. Victor and the vice president for research are given large salary increases and accolades by the university. Is this appropriate? If not, why not?

7.14 Drs. Sterling and Crystal at Research University have been collaborators for a number of years. Each is funded as a principal investigator, with the other as co-investigator, from federal agencies. Drs.

Sterling and Crystal develop strong differences, largely of a personal nature. Dr. Sterling, who is more senior, believes that she "owns" the data and experimental materials derived from the collaboration. Dr. Sterling takes steps to deprive Dr. Crystal of access to the materials. Dr. Crystal appeals to the research administrator of Research University to intervene. The research administrator calls Dr. Sterling and Dr. Crystal together and asks them to "work it out." Drs. Sterling and Crystal cannot reach agreement and Dr. Crystal decides to leave Research University. Dr. Sterling charges Dr. Crystal with intent to remove research materials from Research University without authorization. These accusations are brought to the attention of the federal funding agencies. You are asked to conduct an inquiry. How do you proceed?

7.15 Research University has an umbrella grant from Chemical Corporation. Chemical Corporation dominates the world market in chemical pesticides, herbicides, and rodenticides. Chemical Corporation provides a multimillion dollar grant which Research University uses to support promising research, especially in synthetic chemistry. Dr. Underwood, a microbiologist, has developed a promising biopesticide. Chemical Corporation is not interested in developing this biological product. Dr. Underwood identifies a major agribusiness company that may be interested in funding the development work. Dr. Underwood invites scientists from the agribusiness company to visit his laboratory. Chemical Corporation objects, on the grounds that this violates the provisions of the exclusive agreement between Research University and Chemical Corporation. The research administrator of Research University agrees, but arranges for Dr. Underwood to meet the scientists from the agribusiness company off campus. Is this an appropriate solution?

REFERENCES

1. **Anderson, R. E.** 1990. The advantages and risks of entrepreneurship. *Academe* **6(5)**:9–14.
2. **Association of American Medical Colleges.** 1990. *Guidelines for Dealing with Faculty Conflicts of Commitment and Conflicts of Interest in Research,* p. 18. Association of American Medical Colleges, Washington, D.C.
3. **Barinaga, M.** 1992. Confusion on the cutting edge. *Science* **254**:616–619.
4. **Bourke, J., and R. Weissman.** 1990. Academics at risk: the temptations of profit. *Academe* **76(5)**:15–21.

5. **Bradley, S. G.** 1987. Ethics and intellectual integrity in academia. *SIM News* **37(3):**6–7.
6. **Bradley, S. G.** 1988. University / industry relations and technology transfer. *SIM News* **38:**15–17.
7. **Bradley, S. G.** 1990. Conflicts of interest and conflicts of effort: two distinct afflictions of the academy. *SIM News* **40:**5–7.
8. **Cahn, S. M.** 1986. *Saints and Scamps: Ethics in Academia*, p. 112. Rowman & Littlefield, Totowa, NJ.
9. **Chen, P. S., Jr.** 1992. The National Institutes of Health and its interactions with industry, p. 199–221. *In* R. J. Porter and T. E. Malone (ed.), *Biomedical Research: Collaboration and Conflict of Interest*. The Johns Hopkins University Press, Baltimore.
10. **Cooper, T., and M. Novitch.** 1992. The research needs of industry: working with academia and with the federal government, p. 187–198. *In* R. J. Porter and T. E. Malone (ed.), *Biomedical Research: Collaboration and Conflict of Interest.*The Johns Hopkins University Press, Baltimore.
11. **David, E. E., Jr. (Chairman, Panel on Scientific Responsibility and the Conduct of Research).** 1992. p. 67–79. *In Responsible Science: Ensuring the Integrity of the Research Process*, Vol. I, Ch. 3. National Academy Press, Washington, D.C.
12. **Dustira, A. K.** 1992. The funding of basic and clinical biomedical research, p. 33–56. *In* R. J. Porter and T. E. Malone (ed.), *Biomedical Research: Collaboration and Conflict of Interest*. The Johns Hopkins University Press, Baltimore.
13. **Gillis, A. M.** 1992. The unwilling expert. *BioScience* **42(3):**160–163.
14. **Grinnell, F.** 1987. *The Scientific Attitude*, 2nd ed., p. 101–130. Guilford Press, New York.
15. **Kreiser, B. R.** 1990. On preventing conflicts of interest in government sponsored research at universities, p. 83–85. *In AAUP Policy Documents and Reports*, 7th ed. American Association of University Professors, Washington, D.C.
16. **Kreiser, B. R.** 1990. Faculty appointment and family relationship, p. 116. *In AAUP Policy Documents and Reports*, 7th ed. American Association of University Professors, Washington, D.C.
17. **Marshall, E.** 1992. When does intellectual passion become conflict of interest? *Science* **257:**620–621.
18. **Morgan, H. M.** 1990. Pickled in brine: the possible costs of speculation. *Academe* **76(5):**22–26.
19. **Porter, R. J.** 1992. Conflict of interest in research: personal gain—the seeds of conflict, p. 135–150. *In* R. J. Porter and T. E. Malone (ed.), *Biomedical Research: Collaboration and Conflict of Interest*. The Johns Hopkins University Press, Baltimore.
20. **Roberts, L.** 1992. Science in court: a culture clash. *Science* **257:**732–736.

8 | Ownership of Data and Intellectual Property

Thomas D. Mays

Introduction

Intellectual property is a unique creation of the human mind. It neither has tangible form nor exists apart from the context of the applicable governmental jurisdiction. An observation of a natural phenomenon may not constitute intellectual property. However, commercial utilization or graphic or electronic representation of such a phenomenon would represent intellectual property. In fact, intellectual property only exists as an exercise of a legal right of ownership conferred under statute or common law.[1] The principal types of intellectual property are usually categorized by associating them with the laws covering their use and protection. Such classification yields four types of intellectual property: patents, copyrights, trademarks, and trade secrets.

Author's note: This chapter does not purport, nor was it intended, to provide legal advice. The reader is advised in all instances to seek advice from competent legal counsel in order to ascertain his or her legal rights. There are attorneys trained and qualified to practice the specialty of intellectual property law. The reader is encouraged to obtain legal assistance in order to secure intellectual property rights.

Resource and reference information is presented differently in Chapter 8 as compared with the rest of this book. The references section contains a few citations made in the text, but is generally a reading list to assist the student who needs additional information on the topics discussed here. Endnotes are used to provide specific references, especially in the case of applicable laws, regulations, and policies. Finally, a glossary has been prepared to provide the student with a convenient source of commonly used legal terms.

The protection of intellectual property was guaranteed in 1787 by the United States Constitution, which stated that:

> The Congress shall have Power...To promote the Progress of Science and useful Arts, by securing for limited Times to Authors and Inventors the exclusive Right to their respective Writings and Discoveries...(U.S. Constitution, Article 1, Section 8)

In 1980, a U.S. Supreme Court ruling had an important impact on biotechnological intellectual property. Specifically, the Court ruled in *Diamond v. Chakrabarty* (447 U.S. 303) that nonhuman life forms could be patented if there was an evidence of human intervention in their creation (2).

Every scientist who pursues a course of research using the analytical methodology of observation along with hypothesis formulation and testing follows a long tradition of experimental study. It has been the hallmark of civilization that written records communicate observations, personal impressions, and experimental designs to others geographically and temporally distant to the immediate observer. Through such records, subsequent researchers are able to build upon the work of others. This reflects the central characteristic of scientific discovery; it is a process which builds knowledge incrementally and then pieces that knowledge together in ways that lead to major discoveries. Such discoveries contribute to our understanding of the world and they often can be applied to practical situations leading to advancements that improve the quality of life. This serial advancement in scientific and technological fields has acted as an engine of change that has helped transform societies from agrarian villages to robust industrial centers. While this engine of progress may be fueled by curiosity and personal interest, without a means of engagement, much like the operation of a clutch in an automobile, the progress of science and the useful arts would stall or would have little forward movement. The creators of the U.S. Constitution, in true "serial advancement" fashion, borrowed from and improved upon the experiences of Europe dating back to the 13th century. Specifically, they authorized the protection of ownership of intellectual property by authors and inventors.

Following the U.S. Supreme Court's decision in the *Chakrabarty* case, the last decade has seen an explosion in the commercialization of biotechnology. The certainty of intellectual property ownership in its products has been cited as of utmost importance in preserving competitiveness in the biotechnology industry.[2] Revenues from biotechnology-based pharmaceuticals were estimated to be $1.5 billion in 1989 and $2 billion in 1990.[3]

The potential for biotechnological application makes a basic understanding of intellectual property important in the biomedical disciplines. In this chapter the principles of intellectual property will be discussed, distinguishing between the ethical obligations and the legal rights of ownership in the results of scientific research. We will begin with a discussion of the ownership of research data as a basis for building upon the concepts of intellectual property. Through the use of the case studies the reader is encouraged to consider critically the responsibilities of the scientific researcher under the principles relating to intellectual property rights.

Review of Ownership of Research Data

Research data ownership

Dictionaries typically define data as facts or information which serve as the basis for decisionmaking, discussion and reasoning, or calculation. In the biomedical sciences, intellectual property is almost always grounded in one or more data sets. Thus, we will consider the basic tenets of data ownership before discussing the various categories of intellectual property. The analysis of ownership of research data begins with the question: Who collected the data? However, equally important is the question: Under whose intellectual direction and guidance were the data collected? If the answers to both questions are the same, that person(s) is the tentative owner. The third question that must be asked is whether or not there was a valid obligation to assign the rights in the data to another. This follows the old common law doctrine that workers are entitled to the benefits of their work product, unless they are obligated to give that work product to another, whether in exchange for money, under terms of employment, or under the terms of some rule or law.

When the National Institutes of Health (NIH) of the U.S. Public Health Service awards a research grant to a university, any and all data collected as part of that funded project are owned by the university (commonly called the grantee institution) or by the principal investigator of the grant, depending upon the institution's policy. Thus, all forms of data that are generated as part of an NIH grant-funded research project are the property of the grantee institution. For example, the databooks of the principal investigator, predoctoral and postdoctoral trainees, and other staff members working on the project are the property of the grantee institution. Trainees should not be allowed to take their original databooks with them when they complete their training programs and leave for new positions. However, the removal of copies of original data or databooks may be permitted on a variety of grounds, including duplicative safekeeping and availability of information for manuscript and report writing. Removal of duplicate copies of data should be subject to the approval of the principal investigator. If an investigator were to leave his or her institution during the tenure of an NIH research grant, original data generated as a result of the funded research would still remain the property of the grantee institution. Grants can be transferred from one institution to another when such relocation occurs, but this transfer must meet with the approval of the original grantee institution as well as the NIH. If a principal investigator does not elect to initiate the transfer of the grant from his or her present institution to the new location, then the original grantee institution must petition the NIH to appoint a new principal investigator who would thereafter serve in that capacity.

The scientific community and the public can gain access to original research data obtained as part of federally funded research grants under the Freedom of Information Act (FOIA). This law allows one to request nonclassified information which is available at any agency of the federal government. This is a key consideration in that the data must be in the possession of a federal agency, such as the NIH, a component of U.S. Department of Health and Human Services. Thus, data records are not subject to an FOIA request if they are still in the possession of the grantee institution (i.e., the laboratory of the principal investigator). This situation would be the case for any data that had not been reported to the NIH. Examples of such reported data routinely found in the possesson of a federal granting agency would be those contained in a final report or a progress report which accompanied a new, competing, or continuation grant application. Even if the NIH is in possession of original research data, an FOIA request may be denied if the information is classified under a specified exemption (e.g., trade secrets, commercial or financial information, or intrinsically valuable data used to support a patent application, or to support a request to the U.S. Food and Drug Administration [FDA] for approval of a new drug).[4]

The current rule regarding retention of research data provides that the data be retained for three years from the date of the last expenditure report filed with the granting agency. However, the rights to data access of the granting agency exist for as long as the grantee is in possession of these records. For example, if one should retain databooks from an NIH project that ended 17 years previously, the NIH would still have access rights to them throughout that period. Finally, NIH has the right at any time to inspect any records of the grantee which are pertinent to the award "...to make audit, examination, excerpts, and transcripts."[5] Such regulations for data retention may vary from agency to agency (e.g., public funding agency, private foundation). Principal investigators should always be aware of the pertinent rules and regulations which are applied by their funding sources.

Ownership is in reality an exercise of a property right (i.e., who is able to exert control over the data, at what times, and under what conditions). As in the exercise of any property right, the ownership is dependent on the context of the property. The context of the property in turn depends on how one protects the data and this is defined by intellectual property law.

Legal forms of protection of research data

The United States and many other countries recognize four specific forms of intellectual property for which legal protection is available to the owner. These include: trade secrets, trademarks, copyrights, and patents. The current body of laws providing for ownership or the exercise of property right over these forms of intellectual property have developed over the past 200 years. Under the federal system of government in the United States, the states exercise primary jurisdiction over enforcement of trade secrets and, to an extent, share jurisdiction with the federal government over trademarks and copyrights. It should be noted that the Copyright Act of 1976 provided that federal law would exclusively govern the protection and enforcement of almost all copyrights.[6,7] Patent law has been the exclusive purview of the federal government following the passage of the Patent Act of

1790.[8] While the original colonies granted patents (and some granted copyrights), federal law quickly replaced that of the various states.[9]

Trade Secrets

A trade secret means information, including a formula, pattern, compilation, program, device, method, technique, or process that:

> (i) derives independent economic value, actual or potential, from not being generally known, and not being readily ascertainable by proper means by other persons who can obtain economic value from its disclosure or use and
> (ii) is the subject of efforts that are reasonable under the circumstances to maintain its secrecy.[10]

In other words, a trade secret is information that is not publicly known, but that confers an economic value upon its owner *and* its owner takes reasonable steps to maintain the information as secret. The protection of trade secrets is governed by individual state laws, not federal laws.[11] Legal protection is founded upon principles of contract law and civil misappropriation, but does not cover unauthorized use *per se*. However, legal action can be taken against someone who fails to keep the secret as obligated under contract or a fiduciary relationship or against someone who obtains the secret illegally.[12] A Federal Trade Secrets Act provides criminal penalties for a federal employee who discloses without permission information that concerns or relates to trade secrets of the U.S. government.[13]

For information to qualify as a trade secret, the courts, in actions brought for infringement, have based their decisions on such issues as: (1) the information was not readily available by independent research; (2) the information must have been used in business operations; and (3) the information provided a competitive advantage. Other issues used by the courts in determining the status of a trade secret have included the cost of developing or acquiring the trade secret, who within the business knows the trade secret, and what the business has done to ensure that the information remains secret. However, independent research and "reverse engineering" approaches have been determined to be legitimate means to obtain trade secret information.

Unlike other forms of intellectual property, there is no expiration data for a trade secret. It is in force as long as the information remains secret. This imposes a significant burden upon the owner to take reasonable precautions to ensure that trade secrets do not become publicly known. For example, the recipe for the Coca Cola® brand soft drink has been maintained for many years as a trade secret. However, the moment the company fails to maintain the information as a secret and the information becomes public, the owners will lose the protection of the trade secret.[14] Trade secrets may be assigned or licensed to other parties in the same manner that any other form of intellectual property may be sold or leased. Such arrangements require that the recipient be legally bound to keep the information secret.

Sophisticated and powerful chemical, physical, and biological analytic procedures make the use of trade secrets impractical, especially in the biomedical and biotechnological industries. It would be difficult, if not impossible, today to maintain a genetic cell line, sequence, or other biological composition as a trade secret. Unlike purely chemical compositions, many biological materials have the unique ability to replicate faithfully *in vivo* (e.g., cell line propagation) of *in vitro* (polymerase chain reaction amplification of DNA sequences), thus lending themselves to analysis in ways that can yield secret information. In short, trade secret protection for most biotechnological intellectual property is impractical because of the resolving power of modern analytic technology.

Trademarks

Trademarks embody pictures, sounds, writings, devices, or objects that allow the owner to identify and distinguish some idea, concept, service, or product from those of a competitor.[15] Trademarks protect an idea that conveys the goodwill or reputation of a product or service of the owner. Consumers often rely upon trademarks to know what they can expect if they buy the product or service. This affords a degree of predictability in commerce which is important to business. A related mark is the service mark which serves the same purpose as a trademark but denotes a service rather than a product. Trademarks may be registered at both the state and federal levels. Alternatively, a trademark can be used without any type of legal registration; however, enforcement against an infringer of the mark may then be limited.

Federal trademark registrations are issued by the U.S. Patent and Trademark Office (PTO) for a fee upon the filing of an application by applicant and search conducted by the PTO. Trademark registration lasts for 10 years, but can be renewed indefinitely for 10-year periods (with fees and the filing of an application). Foreign trademark protection must be sought separately in the foreign jurisdiction in which protection is desired. The unauthorized use in commerce of a mark (trademark or service mark) owned by a first party may constitute infringement by a second party if the latter's use creates a likelihood of confusion as to the source of the goods bearing the mark. The courts have considered various defenses to an action against an infringer, including (1) whether or not there was a likelihood of confusion, (2) whether the mark was valid, (3) whether the use was authorized, and (4) whether the mark was merely a descriptive term.

Copyrights

A copyright protects the *expression* of an idea but it does not protect the idea itself. In other words, a copyright protects the *presentation* of an idea, thought, or fact. A copyright does not protect your ideas or other valuable information which you choose to express in some tangible form. Anyone can use your ideas even if they're protected by copyright. In order to copyright something, it must be reduced to a tangible form; you must be able to touch it in order to copyright it. Work to be copyrighted must be fixed in some type of tangible medium. This includes material that must be accessed in some way with the assistance of a machine (e.g., audiotapes, videotapes, and computer diskettes).

A copyright comes into existence the instant the author's words or actions are rendered into some tangible form. Although formal action beyond this is not needed, it is recommended that appropriate forms be filed with the U.S. Copyright Office. In addition, payment of a small fee and deposit of the work with that office are necessary. Copyright works produced after 1977 by individual authors are protected for the life of the author plus an additional 50 years.[16] Copyrighted works created on a "work for hire" basis (see below; employee's creation, but assigned as work by employer) are protected for 75 years from the date of publication or 100 years from the date of creation (whichever comes first).[17] Copyrights on material copyrighted prior to January 1, 1978, were in force for 28 years after initial registration; these were renewable for an additional 47 years.

What may be copyrighted falls into two categories: original works and derivative works. Original works include all forms of tangible expression created independently by the author and not copied from any previous work. An original manuscript prepared on your research findings which contained text, figures, and tables is a good example of an original work. Derivative works would include those works created by the author while relying upon other works, but does not include the mere copying of those works relied upon. As an example here, consider a review article prepared containing numerous and previously published tables and figures from the literature, along with the derivative author's original text interpreting, explaining, or discussing the published literature.[18] Copyright permission would have to be sought and granted to use the figures and tables, but as expressed in your manuscript they would be covered by the copyright protecting your review article. Similarly, your review might discuss the research findings of several papers of others by paraphrasing their writings. This is not a copyright infringement. Moreover, your new written expression of their ideas is copyrighted in your writing.

It is important to distinguish the requirement of *originality* for copyright purposes over the requirement of *novelty* for patent purposes. Work that comprises material that is entirely in the public domain cannot be copyrighted (e.g., common mathematical tables, calendars).[19] The U.S. Constitution provides that only an author is entitled to secure copyright protection. The courts have reasoned that authorship conveys a requirement of originality. The copyright statute similarly provides protection only for *original works of authorship.*[20] While originality may appear to be the same as novelty, "originality means only that the work owes its origin to the author, i.e., is independently created, and not copied from other works."[21] This requirement is in contrast to the prerequisite of novelty for the patenting of an invention. All inventions to be patentable must be novel; that is, the invention must not have been known or used by others in this country nor have been patented or described in a printed publication in this or a foreign country.[22] The requirement for originality is not as rigorous or high a standard as for novelty.[23] The copyright originality requirement is not as difficult to satisfy as the patent requirement of novelty. Because originality is easier to meet, the validity of a copyright based upon the work's originality is easier to defend than the validity of the patent grant based upon the invention's novelty.[24] Conversely, the proof of copyright infringement is more arduous and requires evidentiary showing of not only substantial similarity but also the act of copying.[25]

Consider the following example which invokes the principles of originality and novelty. Laboratory technician Smith creates a computer software program that calculates the half-life of radioisotopes and monitors the inventory of those isotopes in storage using data from a scintillation counter. Ms. Smith's intellectual property could be patented *and* copyrighted. The copyright protection would cover the actual written program (not the idea). The patent would protect the concept of calculating radioisotope half-life and inventory by using the scintillation counter data. The originality of the software would be easily established, since the concept originated from Smith. The novelty of Smith's invention may not be so easily satisfied if another had published a similar (but not the same) invention that used the same elements or components of Smith's invention. If a copyright and patent were each granted to Smith, the validity of the copyright would be difficult to challenge unless the challenger provided evidence of Smith's having copied the work of another. However, the challenge to the validity of the patent may not be as difficult if a challenger were to provide the written description of another's invention that used the same elements or components as Smith used and claimed in her patent.

The owner of a copyright has exclusive rights over reproduction, distribution, sale (or other transfer), and, if appropriate, public performance of the work. The copyright owner also may authorize others to do the same. Copyright is explicitly indicated by the symbol © along with the year of publication or creation. The word "copyright" can be substituted for or used in addition to the © symbol. The author's name should appear along with this indication, if not obvious elsewhere on the work. Indicating copyright in this manner is recommended (but not required) even for unpublished work. Language indicating restrictions is frequently included. Examples of such restrictive language include the following.

- *Copyright © 1991 by John Smith. All rights, including the right of presentation or reproduction in whole or in part in any form are reserved.* This would have special meaning for a work of drama, for example. Even one scene from the play could not be performed publicly without permission from the author.
- *Copyright © 1992 by John Smith. All rights reserved. No part of this publication may be reproduced, stored in a retrieval system, or trans-*

mitted in any form or by any means, electronic, photocopying, re-cording or otherwise without the prior written permission of the publisher and authors. This language speaks to the prohibiting of electronic scanning (or retyping) of material into an electronic format which could be accessed by computer.

Coauthors own the copyright on their part of the work. If partitioning of this sort cannot be plausibly done, then the authors are each equal co-owners of the copyright. They must let each other use the work, but it cannot be licensed to another party without the permission of all of the others. Of course, as with any property right, the true owner(s) may assign his or her rights to another. However, assignment may not be required, if the work constitutes a work for hire. A work for hire is that work prepared by an employee within the scope of his or her employment.[26] Where the employer is the hiring party and the employee has created a specifically assigned work within the scope of employment, the employer will own the copyright. Alternatively, work may be prepared on a special order, commission, or contractual basis and such work is also considered work for hire. In this case, certain requirements must be met. Specifically, a written agreement must exist which provides that the copyright will vest in the hiring party.[27] Furthermore the work must fall into one of nine categories. These include works or writings prepared as (1) a contribution to a collective work, (2) an audiovisual work (e.g., a motion picture), (3) a translation, (4) a supplemental work (i.e., something written to accompany a primary work such as a book foreword), (5) a compilation, (6) a textbook intended for instructional use, (7) a test, (8) answer material for a test, and (9) an atlas.

If an employee is assigned to write an instruction manual for a company instrument, then the copyright belongs to the employer. If, however, the employee writes such a manual without being asked or specifically assigned, then the employee owns the copyright. One academic institutional intellectual properties policy affirms this in the following way: "Assigned duty is narrower than 'scope of employment,' and is a task of undertaking resulting from a specific request or direction. The general obligation to engage in research and scholarship which may result in publication is not an assigned duty. A specific direction to prepare a particular article, laboratory manual, computer program, etc., is an assigned duty" (Intellectual Properties

Policy, Virginia Commonwealth University, Richmond, 1988). Thus, in the context of this language, faculty who prepare original articles on their research findings hold the copyright to such material. When accepted for publication, the author(s) usually assigns the copyright to the publisher of the journal in which it will appear. The NIH and funding agencies in general encourage the publication of research results. The NIH specifically provides that appropriate material created under a grant may be copyrighted by the grantee. In practice, this usually means the principal investigator (and any coauthors) hold the copyright. However, as with ascertaining any legal right, competent legal counsel should be sought in order to understand the effect of all applicable laws and regulations.

Current copyright law provides that *fair use* of copyrighted material will not constitute an act of infringement. An individual may copy from a protected work as long as the value of the work is not diminished and such activity is nonprofit in nature. Fair use activities must be related to (1) criticism, (2) news reporting, (3) teaching, or (4) research or scholarship. Other considerations of fair use include the nature of the work, the quantity and substance of the material being copied as compared with the copyrighted work as a whole, and the possible effect of such use on the potential market for the copyrighted material. Photocopying an article from a scholarly journal for your personal (nonprofit) use is generally recognized as a fair use practice. On the other hand, preparing a compendium of photocopied chapters from several textbooks for use in a graduate course and distributing such documents at a fee to cover the copying costs would likely represent copyright infringement. Such use could be reasoned to diminish value (i.e., students wouldn't buy the books). Thus, the market for the books would be negatively affected. Similar arguments can be made for the photocopying and use of articles from serial publications. Indeed, court rulings have been clear in finding copyright infringement, where one who does not hold the copyright and, without permission of the copyright holder, distributes photocopied compendia of those works as well as third-party copying and distribution of serial publication articles.[28] The interpretation of fair use under the above-mentioned criteria holds that the copying and use be of a personal (nonprofit) nature; that is, articles are copied by the individual who intends to use them under one of the categories related to fair use.[29]

Computer software applications are covered by copyright law. Inspection of program diskettes or accompanying literature will reveal program copyright information. Usually commercially available software is marketed under a so-called *end user's* agreement. Such agreements between you and the software seller provide that you observe copyright law as it pertains to the computer program. Their language usually indicates that the software is being issued to you under a limited, nonexclusive license. This always means you cannot electronically copy the program and provide it to other individuals for their use under any circumstances. Transfer of the software or documentation in whole or in part to another party is often explicitly prohibited. In some cases such agreements specify the conditions for personal use of the software. For example you might only be able to install the program on no more than two of your personal computers. Some software is marketed under agreements called site licenses. This commonly applies to educational and business institutions and involves the authorization of multiple users for a software program. In this case the license is made to the institution and the individual agrees to honor the copyright that protects the software. Site licensed software can be used only at the institution which holds the license. So-called *copy protected* software makes the unauthorized use of software difficult, if not impossible. Copy protection may be part of the software system itself or may involve a hardware device that is sold with the program. Such protection prevents copying or use of the software on machines other than the one on which initial installation took place. Copy protection is used by some manufacturers for specialized or costly programs. However, the vast majority of contemporary software packages do not come with significant copy protection. Thus, users of such software are entrusted with ensuring the appropriate legal operation of purchased programs. Transgressions of computer software copyrights are morally and legally wrong and they can have negative effects on software manufacturers. Disregard for software copyright protection can have devastating effects on small or start-up companies which market computer programs.

Patents

The term "patent" is derived from the Latin *patens* meaning "to be open."[30] This term refers to the royal grants of the British monarchy which were "letters open" or *litterae patentis*. The early British patents granted during the 14th through 16th centuries were in fact royal grants of monopoly in a specific field or for a specific field or for a specific product. A corrupt practice of selling royal grants for tribute brought such patents into disrepute.

The modern patent is a grant by a national sovereign government to an applicant for a specific period of time during which the grantee has a legal right to exclude others from making, using, or selling his or her claimed invention in exchange for the grantee's providing a full disclosure as to how the invention may be made, may be used, or functions. This is the classic example of the *quid pro quo* (this for that), a contractual exchange between parties. One party is the sovereign, acting on behalf of society, who provides this period of exclusivity to the second party, the patentee, in exchange for the patentee's providing a full disclosure of novel, nonobvious, and useful inventions. This exchange is viewed as one of the most powerful forces for advancing the technological basis of a nation's economy. All developed nations have national patent statutes and are signatories to international patent treaties.

A patent is governed by explicit law. The United States patent law can be traced to legislation presented before the first session of the First Congress.[31] Current U.S. patent statutes are the product of several major revisions and recent amendments.[32] Under U.S. law, a patent grants an individual (inventor) or group of individuals (co-inventors) the legal right (personal property right) for a period of 17 years to exclude all others from making, using, or selling the invention as claimed.[33] The term for a utility patent or a plant patent is also 17 years.[34] If a patent claims a composition of matter or process for using a composition of matter that has been subjected to a regulatory review by the FDA, the term of the patent may be extended up to 5 years beyond the original 17-year term.[35] Design patents have a term of 14 years.[36]

In return for this property right, the inventor provides full and complete instructions regarding the claimed invention: how to make or use it, its useful purposes and, to an extent, how it functions. So a patent is a reward for disclosing something of social value to the public. The law states that:

> Whoever invents or discovers any new and useful process, machine, manufacture, or composition of matter, or any new and useful improvement thereof, may obtain a patent therefor, subject to the conditions and requirements of this title.[37]

This law is specific to individual countries, but there is much interest in "harmonizing" patent statutes globally. Patent protection is guaranteed only in the country where the patent has been issued. A U.S. patent on a specific invention does not preclude others from making, using, or selling the invention in Japan, for example.

Contrary to common thinking, under the patent statute, a patent does not give someone the right to make, sell, or practice the invention. It simply permits the inventor to *exclude others* from making, selling, or using the invention. However, common law provides a right to the inventor to practice his or her invention. This right may be dominated by patents held by others. For example, a patent claiming the use of a specific plasmid for the expression of any gene could dominate a patent claiming the use of that vector for the expression of a specific gene. In such a situation, the parties involved would need to cross-license with one another to practice their own invention or risk an infringement action. Because a patent is considered personal property, it can be sold or transferred (assigned) to another or it may be rented (licensed) in whole or in part for the full or partial term of the patent.

To obtain a patent in the United States, one files a patent application with the PTO in Washington, D.C. (the office complex is physically located in Crystal City, Virginia). Prosecution of a patent generally takes from one to several years. In some fields of technology, particularly biotechnology, it may take from three to five or more years before the patent is granted. Patent applications may be prepared and prosecuted before the PTO by registered patent attorneys or registered patent agents. While the inventor is always entitled to prepare and prosecute on his or her own behalf, no one else may represent the inventor before the PTO unless they are admitted to practice before the PTO. The law states that: "Whoever, not being recognized to practice before the United States Patent and Trademark Office, holds himself out or permits himself to be held out as so recognized, or as being qualified to prepare, or prosecute applications for patent, shall be fined not more than $1,000 for each offense" [35 U.S.C. § 33 (1984 and Suppl. 1993)]. The requirement for patent attorneys or agents to be registered by the PTO is to ensure that only qualified practitioners represent inventors. Patent prosecution procedures are highly regulated with a myriad of rules, regulations, and deadlines. The failure to meet a deadline may cause the applicant to lose his or her right to obtain a patent. Generally, in the field of biotechnology, an uncomplicated patent application prepared by a law firm may cost from $10,000 to $20,000. Submission of a patent application is no guarantee, however, that a patent ultimately will be issued.

The United States, the Philippines, and Jordan operate under a "first to invent" policy.[38,39] Patent prosecution and litigation is based on who can demonstrate that they were the first to invent. Most countries operate under a "first to file" system where patents are awarded and litigated based on who files the application first.[40] There is international interest in harmonizing the national patent laws to provide the same standard throughout the world. However, in the United States, there is a long-standing tradition of granting the patent to the individual who invents first.

A compromise appears to be under consideration that would permit "prior user rights" for companies or individuals who have developed and used patentable products or technology but were not the "first to file." However, this proviso would not help university researchers, since most inventions are not commercially practiced in that environment. Instead, universities usually license their patents to companies and prior use rights cannot be transferred to licensees. Current patent law amendments in this area are being argued by some as having severe negative effects on universities.

The types of subject matter that can be patented include processes, machines, products, or composition of matter. Patents can also be sought and obtained for modifications or improvements to any of the above. These types of subject matter may be patentable under a utility patent. Design patents, on the other hand, would provide protection for any new, original, and nonobvious design for a product (e.g., a new automobile body). Any new and distinctive variety of plant, asexually produced (excepting plants of the tuber-propagated family or plants propagated by seed), is patentable subject matter under a plant patent. Sexually reproduced plants and tuber- or seed-propagated plants can be registered by the U.S. Department of Agriculture under the Plant Variety Protection Act.[41]

Subject matter that may be patentable must also be useful, new or novel, nonobvious, and reduced to practice. Reduction to practice must entail either the actual reduction to practice by the creation of a working model (which is operable) or the constructive reduction to practice by the filing of a patent application that provides a comprehensive description enabling one "skilled in the art" to practice the claimed invention. Inventorship of patentable subject matter requires both the conception and the act of reduction to practice. The inventor(s) of an invention who applies for and receives a patent is recognized as the patentee or patent owner; his or her rights under a patent are considered personal property rights and are assignable.

In the absence of a written agreement to the contrary, the patentee owns the patented invention. The employer may obligate assignment of invention rights if the employee is hired to specifically perform research and invent. Under the "shop right" state laws, the employer may own a personal, nontransferable, royalty-free nonexclusive license to the patent *if the employee used the employer's time, materials, or facilities* in the course of inventing. The scope of the shop right is determined from the nature of the employer's business, character of invention, and circumstances of its creation.

The point in time to file a patent should be as soon after the invention is actually reduced to practice or as soon as the inventor is able to provide the full and complete disclosure that is required to achieve the constructive reduction to practice. In the United States, the applicant is permitted to file an application *within* one year of the first disclosure (publication of scientific paper or, in many cases, presentation before a public meeting). However, publication or public disclosure will most likely result in the loss of foreign patent rights, unless a patent application is filed prior to the disclosure. A filing in the U.S. PTO can protect the foreign patent rights if a subsequent foreign patent application(s) is filed within one year of the U.S. filing.

Research sponsored under a federal funding agreement (grant, cooperative agreement, or most contracts) that gives rise to an invention can become the property of the funded nonprofit organization or small business ("contractor"), if the contractor elects to take title to the subject invention and notifies the funding federal agency.[42] When the contractor elects title, it (1) is required to periodically report to the federal agency on the utilization of inventions, (2) is required to place a notice in the patent specification (description) as to the federal support, and (3) must provide a share of the royalties of any licensed subject invention to the inventor and utilize its royalties for scientific research or education. In the event that the contractor declines to elect title to the subject invention, the federal agency determines whether it wishes to elect to take title. If the federal agency declines to elect, the inventor may elect to take title, subject to the federal agency's approval.

The first step to the preparation of filing a patent application is for the inventor to file an Invention Disclosure with the inventor's employer or patent attorney. This is key to securing protection of intellectual property in a patent. Invention disclosure forms vary from institution to institution. The scope of information required by such documents (see below) is exemplified by the information required on the invention disclosure used at Virginia Commonwealth University (Office of Sponsored Programs, Virginia Commonwealth University, Richmond, VA 23298).

The Invention

1. Title of Invention:
2. Attach a concise description of the invention, which should be sufficiently detailed to enable one skilled in the art to understand and reproduce the invention, and should include construction, principles involved, details of operation and alternative methods of construction or operation. Attach drawings, photos, manuscripts, sketches that help describe the invention. Is it a new process, composition of matter, a device, or one or more new products? It is an improvement to, or a new use for, an existing product or process?
3. What is novel or unusual about this invention? How does it differ from present technology? What are its advantages?
4. What is the closest technology currently available, upon which this invention improves?
5. What disadvantages does this invention have? How can they be overcome?
6. What uses do you foresee for the invention, both now and in the future?
7. Has any commercial interest been shown in the invention? Please give company and individuals' names, and addresses if available.
8. What other companies, or industry groups, might be interested in this invention, and why?
9. Please comment on any preferences or ideas you have for a good way to commercialize this invention.
10. What additional work is needed to bring the invention to a licensable state? Please estimate time and cost.

Timeliness and Sponsorship

11. Has the invention been described in a "publication" (journal articles, abstracts, news stories, talks)? Please provide details including dates and copies of written material.
12. Do you plan to publish within the next six months? Please provide approximate date, and any abstract, manuscript, etc.
13. Dates of record, demonstrable from lab notebooks, correspondence, etc.

    Earliest conception _____

    First disclosure _____ to whom: _____

    First reduction to practice _____
14. Please list all sources of support contributing to this invention.

Besides the above, information must be provided concerning the inventor(s) (name, address, etc.), including the percentage of the contribution of each inventor to the invention.

It is essential that the inventor maintain a properly kept laboratory notebook. In addition to being crucial to preparing an invention disclosure or patent application, the research laboratory notebook is frequently used in responding to challenges either during the prosecution of a patent or in postpatent litigation. Maynard (7) has proposed some questions to consider relating to whether or not to file a patent application. Many of these questions can be simply answered by examination of the laboratory notebook. They include:

- What is the nature of the invention?
- When was the invention made and where is the experiment recorded?
- Has the invention been disclosed publicly?
- What is known about the prior work in the field?
- How complete are the data?

Kanare (6) lists additional important points of laboratory notebook writing relating to invention disclosures and patent applications. The conception of an invention that follows from work should be clearly stated. This should be done in a way that documents your own work and compares it to prior work and knowledge in the field. Your laboratory record keeping needs to document that you have worked diligently to reduce your invention to practice. To do this, you must demonstrate that you have worked on your invention continuously. In other words, at no point did you set it aside or abandon it. Having your work witnessed by someone who understands it provides important evidence both in the filing of a patent and in postpatent litigation.

Case Studies

8.1   As is sometimes the case, the student and advisor are not seeing eye to eye. The relationship grows increasingly acrimonious, but the student completes her dissertation and successfully defends it. The student finds a good postdoctoral position and is glad to be moving on. Bitter over the way she believes she has been treated by her advisor, she informs him that she is not going to publish any more of her dissertation work. Further, she informs her advisor that she has copyrighted her dissertation and that he is not allowed to publish any of the work in it either. The advisor is frantic; he received a federal grant to do the work. He needs to show that the proposed work has been carried out by publishing the data in peer-reviewed journals. Yet he is afraid that if he uses any of the data from the copyrighted dissertation he will be sued! What copyright issues and data ownership issues are relevant to this scenario? Imagine you are the faculty member's chair. He comes to you for advice on how to handle this situation. How do you respond?

8.2   A faculty member directs a core laboratory facility at his institution which supplies researchers with custom-made tissue culture media. This is a valuable service which saves investigators time and money. Media can be picked up on four hours' notice and the institution underwrites the facility by paying for the salary of the core lab technician. Thus, the cost of the media is significantly below what can be purchased from commercial suppliers. The rest of the expenses for running the lab (supplies, etc.) are paid for from funds generated from the selling price of the media. The faculty director of the core lab realizes that a clinical facility in his university's medical center is discarding 1-liter glass bottles which had contained tissue culture reagents purchased for use by the clinical lab. He reasons that he can save additional money by washing, sterilizing, and using the discarded bottles to package the tissue culture media sold by his core laboratory. The washing process removes the paper label affixed to the bottle, but does not remove a painted logo used by the company as a trademark. He creates his own labels and affixes the labels on the bottles. The company trademark logo is still visible, however, after the label is in place. Is this a trademark infringement in your view? Would it make any difference if the labels were affixed to the bottles in such a way so as to cover the initial trademark?

8.3 A recently arrived faculty member is setting up his laboratory at an academic institution. He has just assembled his personal computer and has purchased six different software application programs with grant funds. He is preparing to install these programs on the machine when a faculty colleague drops in on him. She suggest that he save time by simply letting her use a portable tape backup system to install the various application software packages on his machine. She says she owns all of the same software and it will take a couple of hours for him to make all of the necessary installation and adjustment settings. She can "dump" all of the same software onto his machine in about 20 minutes. She argues that since he has purchased the identical software for his use, installation of her software on his machine will not be a breach of any copyright or user's agreement. She indicates that while she is at it she will install several other software programs that the faculty member does not own so that he can try them out. She says that the conditions of this "trial" will be that if the faculty member thinks that he will be using the software, he must go out and purchase a copy for himself. Comment on the legal and ethical implications of this scenario.

8.4 A postdoctoral and his mentor have coauthored a paper describing their research results. This paper has appeared as a preliminary report in a copyrighted monograph. One of the figures in this paper is a computer-generated graph that describes data on a series of bacterial growth curves. The postdoctoral and mentor presently are preparing a major paper for submission to a peer-reviewed journal. They both agree that the growth curve data in the monograph article are crucial to the story they're telling in the present manuscript. Accordingly, they decide that this same figure must be included in their present writing. Because they are aware of potential copyright violations, they generate the same figure using different typeface fonts and different line thicknesses for the ordinate and the abscissa. They have decided that since this is not exactly the way the figure appeared in their monograph article, the use of it will not constitute a copyright infringement. They also plan to indicate in their manuscript that this figure has been "adapted from" the one initially published in the monograph article. Comment on what these authors are doing. Do you view it as copyright infringement? If so, are there conditions of modification of tables or figures which would sufficiently change them in a way that avoids copyright infringement?

8.5 Dr. Apple, a researcher working under a National Science Foundation (NSF) grant, is studying the replication of bacteriophage in *E. coli*. Dr. Apple attends a lecture where world-renowned scientist Dr. Ball discusses her studies on the replication of a particularly useful bacteriophage that infects *E. coli*. Dr. Apple requests a sample of Dr. Ball's bacteriophage. Dr. Ball declines to provide a sample, even after several persistent and strongly worded telephone calls from Dr. Apple. Dr. Apple, obsessed with securing Dr. Ball's bacteriophage, has a plan. Dr. Apple writes a letter to Dr. Ball and again requests the material. At the conclusion of the letter, Dr. Apple pleads, "If you insist on denying me this virus, at least give me the courtesy of a written response to this letter." Dr. Ball quickly responds with a one-page, one-sentence response: "Forget it!" After receiving Dr. Ball's letter, Dr. Apple (knowing Dr. Ball's propensity for performing all her working tasks at the lab bench) takes the letter, places it in a blender making a slurry using sterile buffer, and spreads the slurry on lawns of bacteriophage recipient strains of *E. coli*. Soon, Dr. Apple isolates the long-sought strain of the bacteriophage. Were Dr. Apple's actions appropriate? If the bacteriophage were used in a commercial pharmaceutical process and Dr. Ball was employed by the pharmaceutical company, did Dr. Apple illegally obtain a trade secret from Dr. Ball? Should Dr. Apple's actions give rise to an investigation of possible scientific misconduct by the NSF?

8.6 An assistant professor in a biology department is assigned the directorship of an advanced genetics laboratory course to replace a senior faculty member who has just retired and had been the long-standing course director. Over the years, he had compiled an extensive document which the students have used as a laboratory manual. The newly assigned assistant professor proceeds to continue using this "laboratory manual" in the course over the next few years. He modifies and updates it and adds several new laboratory exercises. Following a few more years of evolution, approximately 50% of the laboratory manual has been written *de novo* by the assistant professor. The remaining 50% was written originally by the retired professor but now had been edited by the assistant professor. The assistant professor begins negotiations with a national publisher to develop this laboratory manual as a book. Because of his new writings and his editing of existing material, the assistant professor decides to proceed independently in this venture. What are the copyright implications of this scenario with respect to the assistant professor, the retiring professor, and the university?

8.7 A postdoctoral trainee whose work is funded by a research grant on which her mentor is listed as principal investigator develops a powerful computer algorithm using a commercially available spreadsheet program purchased with the mentor's grant funds. The particular analysis routine which has been developed by the postdoctoral works totally within the spreadsheet application software. It is a sophisticated routine which required many hours of design and testing. Moreover, the postdoctoral has made it available to all members of the mentor's lab and, based on their comments over several months, has introduced many refinements and improvements to the routine. In short, the system can take raw data from enzyme assays and, together with physiological measurements made in animals, statistically analyze data sets and present the results in multiple graphic formats. The application software used for this project was purchased under an academic institutional site license. The software package is copyrighted by the manufacturer. The postdoctoral is considering copyrighting her algorithm before she distributes it to anyone outside the lab. Can she copyright the algorithm? Will this serve any useful purpose? What advice would you give her?

8.8 A faculty member is the director of a two-credit-hour graduate course in molecular genetics. About midpoint through the course, the faculty member is working in the departmental library and notices a three-page, typewritten document on one of the reading tables. Upon inspection, he discovers that this document is a set of typed notes from his October 1 lecture in the molecular genetics course. He reads over the notes and finds them to be an accurate, thorough, and lucid presentation of his lecture. In addition to typed copy, the lecture notes contain computer-generated drawings which represent a compilation of material that he presented using overheads. The notes also contain reproductions of figures from the textbook being used in the course; these appear to have been entered into the document using a scanner. The heading on the first page of this document clearly indicates the lecture title, the date and time, and the faculty member's name. The faculty member then notices the last line of the document, which reads: "Copyright, 1994, James Young." Mr. Young is a student in the class who scored a near perfect grade on the midterm exam in the course. The faculty member approaches one of his own graduate students who is taking the course and asks for an explanation of this material. He learns from his student that Mr. Young has been preparing these class notes for many of the lectures, especially those which cover particularly difficult topics. Mr. Young makes them available on a modest fee basis which includes his cost of duplicating and a small fee-for-service. The student also indicates that only a small number of his classmates in the class have actually purchased the notes for their use. Upon learning all of this information, the faculty member becomes upset and has concerns in several areas. He feels that the student is profiting financially from an unethical practice. He is also concerned that students in the class who use the notes may be benefiting from an unfair advantage. Finally, he is concerned that Mr. Young is guilty of copyright infringement: namely, Mr. Young cannot copyright the faculty member's lecture. Comment on this scenario and the advice that you would give to the faculty member.

8.9 A professor uses a variety of computer software programs in his work-related activities. Because he uses many of these programs in his home office in connection with his scientific consulting activities, he often purchases the software packages with his personal funds; he claims such costs as consulting business-related expenses on his yearly federal tax filing. He often buys upgrades for his software packages. When he acquires such upgrades, he routinely makes a practice of giving the "old" software and its documentation to graduate students or postdoctorals in his laboratory group. He does this under conditions which he defines strictly: the recipient must use the software only on his or her personal computer and may not give copies of it to anyone else. The professor argues that this practice exposes trainees to differing types of software programs and therefore fulfills an educational purpose. Further, he argues that exposure to such software packages is good advertising for software manufacturers; if the trainees like the "old" software, it is likely that they will ultimately buy a copy of the most up-to-date version of the program. Once, when questioned on the legality of this practice, the professor commented that since he had purchased the software, it was his to "give away" if he so desired. He further argued that the restrictions he placed on its use after transfer made such a practice perfectly legitimate. What are your perceptions of the ethical and legal implications of this scenario?

8.10 A university faculty member working in a biochemistry department has developed what she thinks is a patentable idea. Her area of expertise is enzyme catalysis and her idea involves the novel use of a family of enzyme inhibitors in cancer chemotherapy. She holds a grant from the National Cancer Institute entitled "Metabolism in the Neoplastic Cell." The synthesis of this idea has come from her readings outside of what she considers "normal working hours." All of her notes and calculations have been recorded by her at home on a personal computer which she purchased with her own funds for personal use. No experimental work has been necessary to conceive of or to develop this idea. She intends to apply for a patent herself, using her personal funds, and then start a private company to commercialize her idea. Can she rightfully patent her idea in her own behalf? Can her university or the federal government lay any claim to the patent rights in your view? What are the issues of data ownership that impinge on this scenario? Consult the relevant guidelines and policies of your own institution in formulating your response.

8.11 A biochemist from a European country is working as a research associate in a lab at a large university in the United States. The project is supported by funds from the National Institutes of Health and its principal goal is to design, synthesize, and pharmacologically test analogs of a fungal product which has been shown to lower blood pressure in animals. The principal investigator initially assigns some very specific experiments to the research associate but then allows him to work at his own pace. As the work progresses, the research associate embarks on some syntheses that he has come up with on his own. One of these compounds shows very exciting results in lowering blood pressure in animals. The principal investigator is out of the country for three weeks when these results are obtained; moreover, the research associate never told the principal investigator that he was "experimenting on his own," so the principal investigator is totally unaware of the novel compound. The research associate carpools to and from work each day with a law student. He tells the law student about his findings. The law student argues compellingly that the principal investigator will claim ownership over the research associate's discovery and that this would constitute exploitation and intellectual theft. Accordingly, the law student urges the research associate to file an invention disclosure with the university immediately, pointing out the potential for enormous personal financial gain. The law student also suggests that the research associate keep his databooks and related materials on this work at home in a safe place. The law student tells the research associate that the invention disclosure should only list one inventor (i.e., the research associate) since the principal investigator had nothing to do with the conceptualization, synthesis, or testing of this promising new compound. The research associate files the invention disclosure with himself as the sole inventor of the new compound. Comment on this scenario. Is the research associate acting within his rights? Can he legally claim sole inventorship under these circumstances? Assume you are the director of sponsored programs of the university and you have just received the invention disclosure from the research associate. What do you do? Assume you are the principal investigator and have just learned of the entire event from the research associate. Moreover, you learn that the director of sponsored programs has forwarded the invention disclosure to a university committee that will consider its merit in terms of filing a patent application on this discovery. What do you do? Finally, consider the actions of the law student.

Suggested Reading

1. **Barrett, M.** 1991. *Intellectual Property.* Emanuel Law Outlines, Larchmount, NY.
2. **Chakrabarty, A. M.** 1993. Microorganisms having multiple compatible degradative energy-generating plasmids and preparation thereof (U.S. Patent 4,259,444), p. 535–545. *In* J. Davies and W. Reznikoff (ed.), *Milestones in Biotechnology: Classic Papers on Genetic Engineering.* Butterworth-Heinemann, Boston.
3. **Fishman, S.** 1992. *The Copyright Handbook.* Nolo Press, Berkeley, CA.
4. **Foltz, R., and T. Penn.** 1990. *Protecting Scientific Ideas and Inventions.* CRC Press, Boca Raton, FL.
5. **Grisson, F., and D. Pressman.** 1987. *The Inventor's Notebook.* Nolo Press, Berkeley, CA.
6. **Kanare, H.** 1985. *Writing the Laboratory Notebook.* American Chemical Society, Washington, D.C.
7. **Maynard, J. T.** 1978. *Understanding Chemical Patents.* American Chemical Society, Washington, D.C.

8. **Miller, A., and R. Davis.** 1990. *Intellectual Property—Patents, Trademarks, and Copyright in a Nutshell,* 2nd ed. West Publishing Co., St. Paul, MN.
9. **Pressman, D.** 1991. *Patent It Yourself,* 3rd ed. Nolo Press, Berkeley, CA. (Note: A computerized version of this book was marketed by Nolo Press in 1994. It is compatible with Microsoft® Windows™. It contains textual information as well as forms for generating patent applications.)

Glossary

Civil misappropriation: Taking and using of the property of another without permission for the sole purpose of capitalizing unfairly on the goodwill and reputation of the property owner.[43]

Common law: Generally refers to principles of law developed through litigation in the courts, rather than statutes enacted through the legislative process.

Contract law: Subset body of law developed as common law and statute that relates to agreements between parties, including rights and obligations of parties.

Copyright: A property right over intangible intellectual property concerning original works of authorship fixed in any tangible medium of expression.

Derivative work: Work that is compiled by the author from preexisting works; a copyright to a derivative work extends only to that material contributed by the author and not by the preexisting work.[44]

Fair use: Statutory protected form of noncommercial use of work under copyright that includes use of work for purposes of criticism, comment, news reporting, teaching, scholarship and research.

Freedom of Information Act: Statute requiring U.S. government agencies to provide upon request documents in the possession of agency, not otherwise exempted from release under statute [5 U.S.C. § 551 *et seq.* (1977 and Supp. 1993)].

Grantee: Institution, organization, individual or other person designated in a grant; the legal entity to whom a grant is awarded.[45] In the context of federal funding, the party receiving a grant of financial assistance, as provided under 45 C.F.R. Part 74, for grants from the U.S. Public Health Service.

Patent—Design: These patents provide a 14-year period of protection for the ornamental features of an article of manufacture.[46]

Patent—Plant: These patents provide a 17-year period of protection for those plants that the inventor discovers and is able to reproduce asexually, other than tubers (e.g., potatoes).[47]

Patent—Utility: These patents provide a 17-year period of protection for those inventions that are useful, novel, and nonobvious and that constitute a process, machine, manufacture, or composition of matter, or any new improvement thereof; this includes the invention claimed as a drug or claimed as a use of a drug.[48]

Principal investigator: A single individual designated by the grantee in the grant application and approved by the Secretary, U.S. Department of Health and Human Services, who is responsible for the scientific and technical direction of the project.[49]

Statute: An act of the legislature declaring, commanding, or prohibiting something; a law.[50]

Trademark: A distinctive mark that indicates the source of a particular product or service.

Trade secret: A formula, pattern, device, or compilation of information which is used in one's business and which gives one opportunity to obtain economic advantage over competitors who do not know or use it.[51]

Endnotes

1. *Black's Law Dictionary*, 5th ed. (1979), West Publishing Co., at p. 726, col. 2: "Intangibles—Property that is a 'right' rather than a physical object. Examples would be patents, stocks, bonds, goodwill, trademarks, franchises, and copyrights." Also, see "Property, personal, incorporeal," at page 1096, col. 1.
2. *Biotechnology in a Global Economy*, Office of Technology Assessment (October 1991), p. 21.
3. *Idem*, p. 5.
4. 5 U.S.C. § 552(b)(4) (1977 and Supp. 1993).
5. 45 Code of Federal Regulations Part 74.24.
6. Copyright Act of 1976 (P.L. 94-553, 90 Stat. 2541; codified at 17 U.S.C. § 101 *et seq.* (1977 and Supp. 1993)); this act went into effect as of January 1, 1978.
7. See Nimmer on Copyright ("Nimmer"), § 1.01[B], p. 1-7–1-30 (Release No. 29; December 1991).
8. 28 U.S.C. § 1338 (1993).
9. *Walker on Patents*, Deller Ed., Vol. 1, p. 28; 2nd ed., Vol. 1, p. 51, as cited in *Patent Law*, 3rd ed., West Publishing, Choate, Robert A., W.H. Francis and R.C. Collins (eds.) (1987) ("Choate *et al.*"), p. 69, nt. i.

10. Uniform Trade Secrets Act § 1(4) (1985), 14 U.L.A. 286 (Supp. 1987) as cited in *Protecting Trade Secrets, Patents, Copyrights, and Trademarks*, John Wiley & Sons, Dorr, Robert C. and Christopher H. Munch (eds.) (1990) ("Dorr *et al.*"), p. 3, nt. 2.

11. *Idem*, at 8.

12. *Idem*.

13. 18 U.S.C. § 1905 (Supp. 1993).

14. *Op cit*. Dorr *et al.*, p. 9.

15. See generally, Dorr *et al.*, pp. 123–130 and 15 U.S.C. § 1070 *et seq.* (Supp. 1993).

16. 17 U.S.C. § 302(a) (1977 and Supp. 1993).

17. 17 U.S.C. § 302(c) (1977 and Supp. 1993).

18. *Op cit*. Nimmer, § 3.01, at p. 3-2.

19. *Op cit*. Nimmer, see generally, Chapter 2, and specifically, §§ 2.01–2.03.

20. 17 U.S.C. § 102 (1977 and Supp. 1993).

21. *Op cit*. Nimmer, at p. 2-9, citing *Feist Publications, Inc. v. Rural Telephone Service Co.*, 111 S.Ct. 1282, 1287 (1991).

22. 35 U.S.C. § 102 (1984 and Supp. 1993).

23. *Op cit*. Nimmer, at § 2.01[A].

24. *Idem*, p. 2-11.

25. *Idem*.

26. 17 U.S.C. § 101 (1977 and Supp. 1993); also see *op cit*. Nimmer § 5.03[B], p. 5-12–5.32.10.

27. *Op cit*. Nimmer, at 5-32.

28. *Basic Books, Inc., Harper & Row Publishers, Inc., John Wiley & Sons, Inc., McGraw-Hill, Inc., Penguin Books USA, Inc., Prentice-Hall, Inc., Richard D. Irwin, Inc., and William Morrow & Co., Inc. v. Kinko's Graphics Corporation*, 758 F. Supp. 1522, 1526; 18 U.S.P.Q.2D 1437, 1439 (S.D. N.Y. 1991).

29. *Idem*, at 758 F. Supp. 1529; 18 U.S.P.Q.2d 1442.

30. Choate *et al.*, p. 65.

31. *Idem*, p. 75.

32. Current statute is codified at Title 35 United States Code (Supp. 1993) from the Patent Act of 1952. Several bills are pending before the Congress to amend the patent statute to provide, for example: clearer protection of a subject invention from infringement by imported goods; and to clarify that a method of producing a biotechnology invention is not obvious, even if the starting materials are known.

33. 35 U.S.C. § 271 (1984 and Supp. 1993).

34. 35 U.S.C. § 154 (1984 and Supp. 1993).

35. 35 U.S.C. § 155 (1984 and Supp. 1993).

36. 35 U.S.C. § 171 (1984 and Supp. 1993).

37. 35 U.S.C. § 101 (1984 and Supp. 1993).

38. 35 U.S.C. § 135 (1984 and Supp. 1993).

39. *Patents Throughout The World* ("World Patents"), Clark Boardman Callaghan, NY, Jacobs, Alan J. (ed.), Release No. 40, 3 / 92) 1992, at p. J-17 (Release #34, 3 / 90).

40. For example, *op cit.* World Patents, App. B-189 and B-237.
41. 7 U.S.C. § 2402 (Supp. 1993).
42. 35 U.S.C. § 202 (1984 and Supp. 1993).
43. *Black's Law Dictionary,* 5th ed. (1979), West Publishing Co., at p. 901, col. 1.
44. 17 U.S.C. § 103 (1977 and Supp. 1993).
45. 42 Code of Federal Regulations § 52.2(e) (1993).
46. 35 U.S.C. § 171 *et seq.* (1984 and Supp. 1993).
47. 35 U.S.C. § 161 (1984 and Supp. 1993).
48. 35 U.S.C. § 101 (1984 and Supp. 1993).
49. 42 Code of Federal Regulations § 52.2(b) (1993).
50. *Black's Law Dictionary,* 5th ed. (1979), West Publishing Co., at p. 1264, col. 2.
51. *Black's Law Dictionary,* 5th ed. (1979), West Publishing Co., at p. 1339, col. 2.

9 | Genetic Technology and Scientific Integrity

Cindy L. Munro

Introduction

The knowledge and technological advances which have emanated from biomedical research during the past 20 years have been remarkable in a variety of ways. For example, our technological ability to isolate, analyze, replicate, change, and generally manipulate genetic information has jumped several quantum levels since the 1970s. Although recombinant DNA technology began as a research technology, it has quickly been applied to the clinical setting. DNA-based reagents are rapidly emerging as tools with unprecedented power in diagnosing and predicting susceptibility to human diseases. Such diagnostic technologies can be applied at stages that range from conception through adulthood.

The Human Genome Project, which promises to provide genetic mapping and DNA sequence information on the estimated 100,000 human genes, will have immeasurable effects in advancing both DNA diagnostics and therapeutics. It is likely to have applications as yet unimagined. Serious possibilities for abuse of the technology and information exist. The genome project includes a subcommittee to consider the implications for individuals and society. The implications for our view of ourselves and our relationship to other species may be profoundly influenced by knowledge of the human and other genomes.

The isolation and manipulation of genes has launched experimental somatic cell gene therapy and led clinicians to begin to debate the merits and dangers of germ line gene therapy. In addition, genetic manipulation could be used to alter or enhance phenotypes not generally associated with diseases. Interesting questions arise regarding the appropriate uses of genetic manipulation in humans.

Controversy has surrounded the issue of property rights related to genetic information. Some forms of genetic information are patentable. The impact of patenting sequences on the development of genetic biotechnology is an area of much debate.

Genetic Screening and Diagnosis

Detection of gross changes in the morphology or number of chromosomes has been used in postnatal diagnosis of genetic disease since the observation in 1957 that children who had Down syndrome also had three copies of chromosome 21. Prenatal karyotype analysis for chromosomal abnormalities was first reported in 1967 (9), and amniocentesis was clinically available in the early 1970s. Prenatal diagnosis of chromosomal diseases early enough in pregnancy to permit termination quickly became an option available to parents concerned about bearing children free of chromosomal abnormalities.

The development of new techniques in molecular biology has fueled a revolution in genetic testing. Many diseases result from alterations in the DNA which are too small to be seen in a karyotype analysis. Changes in a single base of the DNA may result in formation of an abnormal product in the cell and systemic disease. Examples of diseases which can result from single base changes are sickle cell hemoglobinopathy and cystic fibrosis.

Prior to the advent of technology which enabled direct testing of fetuses for genetic problems, carrier testing was used to provide prospective parents with information about the likelihood of genetic disease in their offspring. This methodology gave prospective parents information which they could use in decisions regarding whether or not they would choose to have children, but did not provide information specific to a particular pregnancy. Information about the genetic health of a fetus can be obtained via a sample of DNA from cells of the chorionic villus at 10 weeks of gestation or from cells in amniotic fluid after 16 weeks of gestation. Results obtained can inform decisions regarding termination of the pregnancy. It is now possible to analyze the DNA of a single cell and to detect changes in DNA as small as a single chemical base. Researchers are exploring the feasibility of isolating fetal cells (for amplification and DNA analysis) from maternal peripheral blood very early in pregnancy; this could provide testing for single gene disorders much earlier in pregnancy without the risks associated with invasive testing such as chorionic villus sampling or amniocentesis.

Advances in DNA amplification, DNA testing, and *in vitro* fertilization technology permit assessment of the genetic health of human blastomeres cultivated *in vitro* before they are selected for implantation. In this relatively new process, ova and sperm are harvested from the parents or donors and conception occurs *in vitro*. After culturing for three days, the fertilized cells have divided to the blastomere stage; each is composed of eight genetically identical totipotent cells. One cell can be removed from each group of eight cells for analysis without disruption of the growth and development of the embryo. DNA sequences of interest can be amplified from the removed cell by polymerase chain reaction (PCR) and the presence of particular sequences associated with disease can be determined. By implanting only blastomeres which are free of the disease sequence, parents can avoid initiating pregnancies which would result in a child with a particular genetic disease and avoid issues of pregnancy termination. Blastomere analysis before implantation has resulted in the births of infants free of cystic fibrosis (16) and Tay-Sachs disease (18). In most cases, parents who are consumers of blastomere analysis technology do not have fertility problems which would prevent natural conception; rather, they choose in vitro fertilization for the express purpose of genetic testing of products of *in vitro* fertilization prior to initiation of a pregnancy.

Initially, genetic testing of adults was a vehicle for informed decisionmaking regarding reproduction. Current applications of genetic testing relate not only to prediction of health of potential offspring but also to disease susceptibility and prognosis in the individual. The current emphasis on primary health care and prevention of disease is congruent with an emphasis on presymptomatic disease testing. In cases where genetic predispositions to disease are known and modifiable risk factors or effective therapies exist, diagnosis of disease prior to the advent of symptoms can prevent the occurrence of disease symptoms. This strategy is illustrated by the well-established newborn screening programs for phenylketonuria (PKU). PKU, a deficiency of phenylalanine hydroxylase inherited in an autosomal recessive pattern, is entirely genetic in etiology, and pathology is entirely preventable. If children with genetic susceptibility to PKU are provided with a diet low in phenylalanine throughout their early development, they grow and develop normally. If, however, phenylalanine is not limited, severe mental retardation and shortened life expectancy result. Since mental retardation in untreated children is evident by age one and is not reversible, it is clearly in the best interests of a child to be diagnosed prior to development of symptoms. Postnatal screening programs, mandated by many state governments, were often based on detection of the presence of phenylalanine by-products in the urine or phenylalanine levels in the blood. Since the gene for phenylalanine hydroxylase has been cloned, it is now possible to test directly and prenatally for the defect. Similar strategies might be available for some adult-onset diseases with a genetic component. For example, dietary or activity modifications to reduce risks of heart disease would be particularly important for individuals who have genes which would predispose them to heart disease.

The use of DNA-based screening for diseases which have a genetic component can pose particularly difficult dilemmas. In most cases, the ability to identify particular genes generally precedes thorough understanding of the implications of presence of a defective gene and effective treatment. It could be argued that providing individuals with knowledge of potential for disease promotes autonomy; however, a person's welfare may or may not be enhanced by knowing that one has a predisposition toward a disease for which there is currently no preventive therapy and no cure. Would it benefit or harm the person to know, years in advance of symptom development, that the future is likely to hold Huntington's chorea, breast cancer, or colon cancer?

Although it may be possible to predict genetic or chromosomal disease, the variability of individuals in disease course and severity complicates the issue of decisionmaking. Clinicians have been able to accurately predict trisomy 21 prenatally since amniocentesis became widely available in the 1970s; it is still not possible to predict for parents from a karyotype whether their fetus who has Down syndrome would grow to be a mildly retarded adult capable of functioning independently or a severely retarded individual who would require extensive and expensive care.

Further complications are posed by the uncertainties of future options. It is not possible to predict what therapies for management or cure of disease may be developed, nor when these therapies will be available to patients. For example, many innovative therapies are currently available for cystic fibrosis, and both life span and quality of life have improved considerably for patients in the last decade. However, these advances were not predictable to clinicians providing prenatal genetic counseling a decade ago.

Quality of life of individuals affected with a particular disease is not predictable by genetic tests. Not only do course and severity of illnesses vary on an individual basis, but individuals at the same level of severity may have very different perceptions of how burdensome the disease is and the degree to which it affects the quality of their lives. This individual variation in requirements for and perception of quality of life may not be recognized by others and may lead to assumptions about what is necessary for a meaningful life. Arguing in favor of the benefits of prenatal diagnosis and selective termination of pregnancy, L. G. Jackson states, "It is intended to relieve suffering and improve health. It is obviously admitted that it would be better to have curative approaches to genetic diseases, or successful treatment approaches if cure is not possible. However, all practicing physicians recognize the incredible burden of chronic diseases and genetic disorders, especially those beginning early in life. The fact that caring parents would wish not to burden their offspring with such extraordinary difficulties simply represents the good attitude of one human being toward another" (19). H. DeRogatis, a nurse who speaks about her own disability, offers a different viewpoint. She says, "Our culture does not reflect the ways in which people with disabilities experience and value our bodies and our lives...I understand that it may be difficult for able-bodied people—particularly those in the health professions—to believe that disability may be experienced as different, not less" (11).

Concerns also exist about the confidentiality and use of genetic information and results of genetic tests. Unlike many other specimens, genetic information can be stored for long periods in the form of a frozen blood sample. This sample provides a source of material which can be analyzed for factors other than what was originally intended and at a time removed from the collection and consent process. It is vital that informed consent be elicited from patients in health care settings and subjects in research settings; those from whom specimens are collected should give express permission for analysis and should be made aware of confidentiality safeguards in storage and future use of the material.

The Department of Defense plans to store a blood sample from each active-duty service member by 1999 and from each reservist by 2005. The DNA in this stored sample would serve as a source of "genetic dogtags," permitting identification of remains. The Department of Defense has provided assurances that this genetic information will not be used for any other purpose. The FBI and some states have demonstrated interest in maintaining samples of DNA as part of penal records for individuals convicted of crimes.

The appropriateness of use of genetic information by employers for preemployment screening or job assignment is debatable. It has been argued by some that screening of individuals for susceptibility to injury in a particular workplace (for example, related to genetic susceptibility to disease related to chemicals in use at the job site) promotes the health of individual workers and reduces job-related morbidity, thus reducing employers' health care costs. Such information about susceptibility might be used in a variety of ways: to counsel employees regarding risks, to institute more careful safeguards against exposure, to guide frequency of health monitoring, to assign jobs, or to influence hiring decisions (8). Public health benefits may also accrue from an ability to identify those who might be more likely to develop a workplace disability which would endanger coworkers or the public. However, genetic information is often erroneously applied and may be discriminatory. Employers may confuse those who carry one allele of a recessive disorder (carriers) with those who have the disease. Treating those who have a genetic predisposition as if they were already ill (or inescapably destined to become ill) can lead to discriminatory practices. One large company was found to be discriminating against persons who had sickle cell trait although the trait had not been shown to be associated with higher workplace disability (12, 25). H. Ostrer et al. (28) examined the application of The Americans with Disabilities Act of 1991 (ADA) to genetic information. Although the ADA does not permit medical testing prior to an employment offer, genetic testing would be permissible as long as all entering employees were required to have the same examination. Tests performed would not have to be related to current job performance but could extend to other conditions which might affect future benefit claims. It is not yet known whether the ADA will provide protection to presymptomatic individuals with genetic predisposition to disability (28).

Discrimination may occur in health, disability, and life insurance coverage as well. In one reported instance, a health maintenance organization attempted to limit postnatal coverage of a fetus whom the parents elected not to abort following a positive genetic test for cystic fibrosis (17). P. R. Billings et al. (3) described 41 separate incidents of discrimination against individuals which occurred "solely because of real or perceived differences from the 'normal' genome." T. H. Murray (25) notes that participation as a research subject in predictive genetic studies may adversely affect access to insurance.

The Human Genome Project

The Human Genome Project intends to provide genetic maps, physical maps, and nucleotide sequence data from the human genome and the genomes of several model organisms. From the initiation of the project in October 1988, approximately 5% of the budget has been directed to consideration of the social, legal, and ethical implications of the project. The information generated by the project will be a valuable tool to researchers in localizing and isolating DNA sequences associated with diseases or other traits. Public access databases have already been developed which permit electronic access to primary data, maps, marker information, and reference information (7). As more specific DNA sequences are associated with particular diseases or other phenotypes, ability to detect genetic predisposition to disease (and attendant problems addressed above) will explode. We will also gain insight into the genetic component of human traits not generally associated with disease.

Advancing knowledge of the genome may fundamentally alter our view of humanity. Investigations regarding genetic influences on behaviors are currently stirring controversies about the extent of choice and responsibility in behavior. Identification of a genetic component to behavior does not predetermine how we will interpret or apply such information. For example, male homosexuality has been linked to a region on the X chromosome (15, 22); how does this demonstration of a genetic component to homosexuality affect or inform our views of homosexual behavior? Provided with the same data (that male homosexuals differ from heterosexual males in a particular genetic region), one might conclude that homosexual behavior is a normal variation in human sexual expression, or that it is an abnormal "disease" allele. Increased information about genetics may lead to either increased acceptance or renewed rejection of particular groups of individuals.

Comparisons of the genomes of humans and other organisms may affect our associations with the larger world. T. H. Murray suggests that in light of examination of our genetic relatedness to other species, "we may reevaluate not only our molecular but also our moral relationship with nonhuman forms of life" (24).

B. M. Knoppers and R. Chadwick (21) suggest that international consensus regarding the ethical problems posed by the Human Genome Project is already developing. They propose that this consensus is based upon the principles of autonomy, privacy, justice, equity, and quality. Although there may be some agreement regarding broad ethical issues related to human genome research, the interpretation and evaluation of specific challenges will likely generate lively debates.

Manipulating Genes

The notion that we may be able to directly manipulate human genetic material and affect changes in the function of genes has been enlivened by the Human Genome Project and advances in molecular biology. Technology which permits direct intervention at the molecular level, coupled with increased knowledge about the location, structure, and function of genes, provides possibilities for changing sequences in order to alter the function of particular genes. Such interventions are currently being explored in somatic cell gene therapy and could also be applied to germ line cells. Current efforts focus on prevention or treatment of diseases, but the same techniques could be applied to alter genes not commonly associated with diseases.

Somatic cell therapy

Somatic cell gene therapy is currently being used in clinical trials. Inherited disorders such as cystic fibrosis are obvious targets for gene therapy. However, somatic cell manipulation has also been proposed as therapy in cancers (10,30), cardiovascular diseases (14), and infectious disease such as human immunodeficiency virus (HIV) infection (13). Different methods for gene delivery are being tested based on target cell typology. For example, in a clinical trial for the treatment of cystic fibrosis, a functional copy of the *CTFR* gene is delivered to respiratory epithelial cells by inhalation of an adenoviral vector carrying the gene (6). Adenoviral vectors do not require active target cell division, making them appropriate vectors for terminally differentiated cells of the respiratory tract. In this case, the therapeutic effect is lost when the treated cells die; this gene therapy provides treatment, but not cure. Retroviral vectors are able to integrate into a chromosome of a target cell, and future generations of that cell will inherit the introduced gene. If the targeted cell is a stem cell, it could provide populations of cells with the introduced gene over a long period of time. In this case, it might be appropriate to speak of the gene therapy as a cure. In somatic cell therapy, alterations introduced affect only the individual recipient of therapy; they are not inherited by offspring of the treated person.

Some somatic cell therapies have been targeted to treating genetic diseases. Gene therapy for single gene recessive disorders requires only gene addition for treatment. Providing the ability to make adequate amounts of a functional gene product results in amelioration of the disease. In 1993, reports of the successful treatment of two young girls with adenosine deaminase deficiency was reported in the media (4,31). Strategies for dominant disorders and multigene disorders will be more difficult. In dominant disorders, disease results not from the absence of a functional gene product but from the presence of an abnormal product. Treatment would be contingent upon ceasing production from the affected gene(s) and might also involve providing a normal copy of the gene if none is present.

A variety of approaches have been suggested to harness gene therapy to the treatment of HIV infection. E. Gilboa and C. Smith (13) classify these approaches as either intracellular immunization or immunological gene therapy. Intracellular immunization involves transfer of genes which inhibit viral replication into hematopoietic cells to reduce spread of HIV within an individual. Immunological gene therapies are designed to enhance the natural defenses of the infected individual.

Genetic manipulation of somatic cells for the purpose of treating or preventing disease poses fewer ethical dilemmas than does manipulation aimed at germ cells or alteration of nondisease genes. W. F. Anderson, a pioneer in gene therapy, states, "There is now a general consensus that somatic cell gene therapy for the purpose of treating a serious disease is an ethical therapeutic option" (1). Although *in vitro* laboratory studies and animal experiments precede all clinical trials, and initial human trials have been encouraging in many gene therapy protocols, it is important to remember that all current gene therapies are experimental. It is important for both clinician researchers and subjects to understand the experimental nature of the work. Apprising subjects of possible risks as well as potential benefits is an essential component of obtaining informed consent. The novel nature of these therapies makes it difficult to anticipate risks. Somatic cell gene therapies may have both immediate and delayed unanticipated complications. Several safety issues are of potential concern in somatic cell therapy. Depending upon the method of gene delivery, family members and those caring for the gene therapy patient may inadvertently be inoculated. Present methods do not permit targeting of genes inserted by retroviral vectors to a particular chromosomal location. Insertion of the introduced gene could theoretically result in a harmful mutation at the insertion site, resulting in loss of a critical cell function or loss of growth control. Regeneration of infectious particles from viral vectors is thought to be unlikely, but is nonetheless a potential problem. There are concerns that an immune response may be generated against target cells following gene therapy. However, the risk to date remains hypothetical; no pathologic events or malignancies have been noted yet in animal or human subjects (14).

Germ line therapy
Manipulation of DNA in germ cells raises additional issues. Manipulations which affect ova, spermatozoa, or totipotent cells such as blastomeres are heritable. Changes made to the DNA in these cells have the potential to affect not only the individual treated but also his or her offspring. Germ line manipulation has been accomplished in mammals and use of genetically manipulated animals is widespread in research. In the production of transgenic mice, for example, the genetic material of an embryonic stem cell is the target. The cell is then cloned and used to establish a lineage of mice carrying the added (or altered) genetic material (5). Feasibility of the techniques has not yet been demonstrated in human cells.

The benefits and risks of germ line gene therapy in humans have been widely debated; for example, the *Journal of Medicine and Philos-*

ophy devoted an entire volume (Volume 16) in 1991 to the ethics of human germ line genetic manipulations. N. A. Wivel and L. Walters (33) recently reviewed mouse model systems for human diseases which might be amenable to germ line therapy, and suggested clinical scenarios for the use of germ line therapy in humans.

Many of the concerns raised in the consideration of somatic cell therapy apply to germ cell therapy as well. Even when restricted to prevention of and therapy for severe genetic diseases, germ cell therapy poses additional questions as well. The potential to do good for multiple potential individuals in a single intervention is great; it would be much more effective to prevent disease in all of the future branches of a patient's family tree than to treat each descendant individually for the disease. This potential to maximize beneficence is attractive to health care providers. However, accompanying the potential for good is a potential for harm. Any untoward effects of germ cell manipulation may also be propagated to the patient's descendants. Concerns have also been expressed regarding the balance of individual autonomy (arguing that decisions about genetic manipulation are best made by the individual involved or parental surrogates) and society (arguing that since germ cell manipulation potentially affects more than the individual and may have far-reaching future effects, society has a legitimate interest in the availability and use of the technology).

Enhancements

The preceding sections addressed manipulation of genetic material of either somatic cells or germ cells in efforts to prevent, treat, or cure disease. Many have argued that genetic manipulations should be reserved for the treatment or prevention of serious disease. W. F. Anderson articulates this view: "Although the medical potential is bright, the possibility for misuse of genetic technology looms large, so society must ensure that gene therapy is used only for the treatment of disease" (1).

Techniques being developed to permit modification of phenotypes associated with disease could be used to modify other characteristics. Such modifications depend upon an exquisite knowledge of the location and operation of genes which is not currently available. The genome project will provide valuable information to spur the research of those interested in traits not currently associated with disease. Speculation about the ramifications of manipulation of the human genome to alter or enhance particular nondisease traits is an active area of discourse.

It is likely that some healthy individuals will seek genetic manipulation. For example, some athletes have sought improvement in their oxygen-carrying capacity by a variety of means. High-altitude training has been used to elevate hemoglobin levels. Blood doping, via removal of blood one month prior to a critical sports event and autotransfusion just before the event, has been used to increase the number of circulating erythrocytes during competition although the practice is prohibited by most organizations governing athletic competitions. Biosynthetic erythropoietin (EPO), developed for the treatment of chronic anemias, is of current interest to some athletes. T. H. Murray (24) reports that EPO has been classified as a performance-enhancing drug by the International Olympic Committee. Those athletes who are willing to use pharmacologic and invasive methods in an effort to improve performance might view genetic manipulation as an additional tool to maximize oxygen capacity.

In the example of EPO, techniques currently being developed for use in treatment of hematologic disease may be appropriated by healthy individuals for the purpose of enhancement. In other instances, individuals may seek cosmetic alterations. Somatic cell gene therapy has sometimes been viewed as an alternative method for producing therapeutic results we would seek from surgery or pharmacologic agents (26). This view of somatic cell gene therapy as equivalent to other therapeutic modalities complicates the issue of cosmetic enhancement. Is genetic enhancement akin to cosmetic surgery? Both pharmacologic agents and surgical methods are used to alter the appearances of individuals who are within the range of normal appearance and function before intervention. We do not limit the autonomy of individuals to undergo cosmetic surgery, except in special circumstances where such surgery might negatively impact physical or mental health. Indeed, many of those who choose current methods for enhancement of appearance experience positive benefits such as an improvement in quality of life and enhanced self-esteem. If techniques can be developed which are relatively safe and effective, similar benefits might accrue to individuals who achieve cosmetic results via somatic cell gene manipulation.

The manipulation of germ line material outside of its use in disease prevention and treatment has generated much controversy. Issues of personal and parental autonomy and of consent are more problematic when changes may affect future generations, particularly when changes are not initiated in response to potential or actual disease. Decisions may have broader societal effects, and the specter of the development of a genetic class system has negative implications. T. Peters states, "The growing power to control the human genetic makeup could foster the emergence of the image of the 'perfect child' or a 'super strain' of humanity; and the impact of the social value of perfection will begin to oppress all those who fall short" (29). Not all agree that use of germ line manipulation to affect nondisease traits will necessarily have a negative effect on individuals or society. It is quite possible that different parents would prefer and select different traits, without a societal trend for some selections to be labeled as preferable by the society as a whole. Arthur Caplan, a noted bioethicist, recently said in regard to germ line manipulation, "The question of whether I should be able to pick blue eyes or brown or tall people or short — I don't think there's anything wrong with that fundamentally" (2).

Genetic Information and Property Rights

Some interesting issues have been raised in regard to ownership of genetic information. D. J. Kevles and L. Hood express a common sentiment when they state, "If anything is literally a common birthright of human beings, it is the human genome" (20). However, genetic material in some forms can be owned; it is patentable and the limits of patent protection are being tested. Intellectual property may be protected by patent. Issuance of a patent provides a statement of ownership of a particular intellectual property and gives the owner the right to exclude others from making, using, or selling intellectual property without permission. Patents in the United States can be issued for any machine, article of manufacture, process, or composition of matter. In addition, the patent subject must be new, useful, and nonobvious.

Compositions of matter must be in a form different from that found in nature; proteins which have been isolated and purified have been successfully patented. The category of composition of matter is not limited to inanimate matter. Patents have been granted for genetically altered microorganisms, plants, and animals (23,27). DNA, as a composition of matter, falls within the definition of patentable material.

It has been argued that the human genetic sequence is not new. But in converting the sequence to a compostion of matter different from that which exists in nature, the sequence does become new. In some cases, cDNA (complementary DNA) is the subject of the patent application. cDNA is constructed using messenger RNA as a template and so does not contain introns; thus, it differs from the sequence of DNA as found in nature and is new. The sequences used to produce human insulin, human erythropoietin, and other biologic pharmaceuticals have been patented. The sequence does not have to correspond to the full length of a gene, nor even to include potential coding sequences. Genetic probes used in detection of genomic sequences and oligonucleotide primers for PCR are potentially patentable. It is not necessary to know the function of a sequence prior to applying for or obtaining patent, so long as the new, useful, and nonobvious criteria can be demonstrated (32).

Issuance of patents for sequences embedded in the human genome is controversial. The patent system was designed to encourage research and development of technology. It provides a reward for a patent owner in the form of the ability to restrict others from using one's intellectual property. When the patented genetic sequence can be used to make a pharmaceutical product such as human insulin or human erythropoietin, or can be used as a diagnostic probe for disease, economic advantages may result. However, there are concerns that the patent process may impede research. Patenting may impose barriers to free intellectual exchange. Although the norms of most scientific disciplines have encouraged free exchange of biological samples and reagents, patents provide holders with the authority to forbid or limit the use of patented materials. Some researchers may delay publication until after patent filing. Informal discourse and synergy between researchers might be adversely affected as well. It is not yet clear whether the patent system will have a measurable positive or negative effect on genetic biotechnology.

Conclusion

Genome and biomedical research have exploded in the past decade, but even more revolutionary developments are on the horizon. Somatic cell gene therapy for a variety of diseases is currently under way. Integration of somatic cell therapies into usual medical practice may not be far distant, and germ line gene therapy is an active area of discussion. Whether gene therapies will be limited to serious diseases or used over the same spectrum of care as current medical and surgical interventions remains an issue. As the Human Genome Project progresses, it is certain to have wide-reaching effects on research and knowledge about our genetic selves. Coupled with the ethical and moral decisions genetic technology poses, legal and economic layers of complexity are added by the potential impact of the patent system. Many issues have been raised in this discussion. Some of the questions which will be most crucial regarding impact of the technology cannot be envisioned at our current level of understanding. Formulating the questions and articulating the issues is a beginning step in preparing to meet the challenges to health care and scientific integrity posed by the expanding area of genetic biotechnology in these contexts.

Case Studies

9.1 The prospects of genetic screening raise interesting and sometimes controversial issues when applied to the family setting. Disclosing information may violate a sibling's right to privacy, but withholding it may cause harm too. How should information discovered by genetic technology in one family member be treated if it could affect other family members as well?

9.2 Consider a diagnostic DNA probe that could provide information on the nature of some types of neoplastic disease. Specifically, the probe in question can determine whether the specific cancer is aggressive or relatively slow growing. Proponents of the clinical use of such a probe argue that it promises to provide important prognostic information and potential guidance toward the effective use of anticancer therapies. Opponents argue that such information is likely to make its way into databases that can adversely affect a patient's ability to secure various types of insurance and in general threaten an individual's right to privacy. Discuss the scientific and ethical implications of this scenario.

9.3 You have been named to a task force of a national biological society of which you are a member. The principal duty of this task force is to develop a position with respect to human genetic diagnostics. This position will be voted on by the entire society. The basic premise being addressed concerns the increasing availability of gene probes that provide the direct or indirect means for the diagnosis of genetic diseases or genetic states which predispose to disease. It is obvious that in many cases such diagnoses involve diseases which cannot be cured, prevented, or even treated. The first meeting of the task force opens with the chairman proposing that the committee embrace the following concept. Specifically, the members of the society should be asked to vote on a resolution that states that no gene probe should be used in a human clinical diagnostic situation involving a disease for which there is not a significant therapeutic intervention that either improves the patient's quality of life or prolongs it. What would be your arguments either for or against this proposal and what is the rationale underlying your arguments? If you feel the proposal has merit but needs modification, articulate the changes that you would like to see made to it.

9.4 As the human genome sequencing project moves forward, certain investigators have been advised by the NIH Office of Technology Transfer to apply for patents covering cDNA sequences derived from the fragments of human genes. Although the ultimate function and specificity of such sequences are not known at present, it is argued that such fragments can be used as probes to eventually locate complete genes. Comment on the intellectual property and ethical considerations of patenting uncharacterized human cDNA sequences.

9.5 A recently enacted state law requires the state's Division of Forensic Science and Investigation to analyze, classify, and store the results of DNA identification characteristics ("DNA fingerprints") from all convicted felons. Thus, blood samples must be taken from felons in order to implement this plan. The results must be maintained electronically in a DNA data bank which is available for criminal investigation. Only 10% of the available blood samples have been processed and DNA data entered when the state police develop a suspect in a series of rape cases. The suspect had been previously convicted and sampled, but his blood has not yet been analyzed, so his DNA pattern is not presently in the data bank. The investigators do not have sufficient probable cause to get a blood sample from the suspect, so they ask that the division's blood samples be processed now and analyzed together with the evidence from the crime scene. Do you think this is this legal? Is it ethical? How should the results be reported in the event of a match? A nonmatch?

9.6 Some argue that the advent of DNA data banks of convicted felons represents an infringement on the constitutional rights to privacy and therefore should be abolished. Would it be appropriate to use such data for research purposes as long as personal identifiers were not released to the researchers?

NOTE: For 9.7–9.10, use the following information to frame discussion. In their book *Genethics* (Harvard University Press, Cambridge, MA, 1990), David Suzuki and Peter Knudtson propose a number of "genethic principles." Comment on the plausibility of the selected principles listed below and discuss relevant issues regarding their implementation in the scientific community and in general society.

9.7 "To grasp many of the difficult ethical issues arising from modern genetics, one must first understand the nature of genes — their origins, their role in the hereditary processes of cells and the possibilities for controlling them."

9.8 "The vast majority of human hereditary differences are polygenic, or involve the interplay of many genes; therefore, it is a dangerous simplification to proclaim a causal relationship between human behaviors and so-called 'defects' in human DNA."

9.9 "While genetic manipulation of human somatic cells may lie in the realm of personal choice, tinkering with human germ cells does not. Germ-cell therapy, without the consent of all members of society, ought to be explicity forbidden."

9.10 "Until we have a better understanding of the extent of genetic exchange between distantly related species in nature, we ought to consider evolutionary 'boundaries' — areas of relatively limited genetic exchange — as at least provisional warning signs of potential danger zones for the casual transfer of recombinant genes between species."

REFERENCES

1. **Anderson, W. F.** 1992. Human gene therapy. *Science* **256**:808–813.
2. Arthur Caplan discusses issues facing the growing field of bioethics. (October 17, 1994.) *Scientist* **8(20)**:12, 25.
3. **Billings, P. R., M. A. Kohn, M. de Cuevas, J. Beckwith, J. S. Alper, and M. R. Natowicz.** 1992. Discrimination as a consequence of genetic testing. *Am. J. Hum. Genet.* **50**:476–482.
4. **Blaese, R. M.** 1992. Development of gene therapy for immunodeficiency: adenosine deaminase deficiency. *Pediatr. Res.* **33**(Suppl.):S49–S55.
5. **Bradley, A., P. Hasty, A. Davis, and R. Ramirez-Solis.** 1992. Modifying the mouse: design and desire. *BioTechnology* **10**:534–539.
6. **Brody, S. L. and R. G. Crystal.** 1994. Adenovirus-mediated *in vivo* gene transfer. *Ann. N. Y. Acad. Sci.* **716**:90–101.
7. **CHLC (Cooperative Human Linkage Center).** 1994. A comprehensive human linkage map with centimorgan density. *Science* **265**:2049–2054.
8. **Council on Ethical and Judicial Affairs, American Medical Association.** 1991. Use of genetic testing by employers. *JAMA* **266**:1827–1830.
9. **Cowan, R. S.** 1992. Genetic technology and reproductive choice: an ethics for autonomy, p. 244–263. *In* D. J. Kevles and L. Hood (eds.), *The Code of*

Codes: Scientific and Social Issues in the Human Genome Project. Harvard University, Cambridge, MA.

10. **Culver, K. W.** 1994. Clinical applications of gene therapy for cancer. *Clin. Chem.* **40:**510–512.

11. **DeRogatis, H.** 1993. A different reflection. *Nurs. Outlook* **41:**235–237.

12. **Fost, N.** 1992. Ethical implications of screening asymptomatic individuals. *FASEB J.* **6:**2813–2817.

13. **Gilboa, E., and C. Smith.** 1994. Gene therapy for infectious diseases: the AIDS model. *Trends Genet.* **10:**139–144.

14. **Goldspiel, B. R., L. Green, and K. A. Calis.** 1993. Human gene therapy. *Clin. Pharm.* **12:**488–505.

15. **Hamer, D. H., S. Hu, V. L. Magnusen, N. Hu, and A. M. L. Pattatucci.** 1993. A linkage between DNA markers on the X chromosome and male sexual orientation. *Science* **261:**321–327.

16. **Handyside, A. H., J. G. Lesko, J. J. Tarin, R. M. L. Winston, and M. R. Hughes.** 1992. Birth of a normal girl after *in vitro* fertilization and preimplantation diagnostic testing for cystic fibrosis. *N. Engl. J. Med.* **327:**905–909.

17. **Holtzman, N. A.** 1992. The diffusion of new genetic tests for predicting disease. *FASEB J.* **6:**2806–2812.

18. Institute rejects offering parents vote on baby's sex, p. B4. (September 3, 1994.) *The Richmond Times-Dispatch.*

19. **Jackson, L. G.** 1990. Commentary: Prenatal diagnosis: the magnitude of dysgenic effects is small, the human benefits, great. *Birth* **17:**80.

20. **Kevles, D. J., and L. Hood.** 1992. *The Code of Codes: Scientific and Social Issues in the Human Genome Project.* Harvard University, Cambridge, MA.

21. **Knoppers, B. M. and R. Chadwick.** 1994. The Human Genome Project: under an international microscope. *Science* **265:**2035–2036.

22. **LeVay, S., and D. H. Hamer.** 1994. Evidence for a biological influence in male homosexuality. *Sci. Am.* **270(5):**44–49.

23. **Murashige, K. H.** 1994. Intellectual property and genetic testing. *In* M. S. Frankel and A. Teich (eds.), *The Genetic Frontier: Ethics, Law, and Policy.* AAAS, Washington, D.C.

24. **Murray, T. H.** 1991. Ethical issues in human genome research. *FASEB J.* **5:** 55–60.

25. **Murray, T. H.** 1993. Ethics, genetic prediction, and heart disease. *Am. J. Cardiol.* **72:**80D–84D.

26. **Nolan, K.** 1991. Commentary: How do we think about the ethics of human germ-line genetic therapy? *J. Med. Philos.* **16:**613–619.

27. **O'Conner, K. W.** 1992. Patenting life. *Cancer Invest.* **10:**61–70.

28. **Ostrer, H., W. Allen, L. A. Crandall, R. E. Moseley, M. A. Dewar, D. Nye, and S. V. McCrary.** 1993. Insurance and genetic testing: where are we now? *Am. J. Hum. Genet.* **52:**565–577.

29. **Peters, T.** 1994. Intellectual property and human dignity. *In* M. S. Frankel and A. Teich (eds.), *The Genetic Frontier: Ethics, Law, and Policy.* AAAS, Washington, D.C.

30. **Sikora, K.** 1994. Genes, dreams, and cancer. *Br. Med. J.* **308**:1217–1221.
31. **Thompson, L.** June 7, 1993. The first kids with new genes. *Time* **141(23):** 50–53.
32. **White, T. J.** 1994. Intellectual property and genetic testing: a commentary. *In* M. S. Frankel and A. Teich (eds.), *The Genetic Frontier: Ethics, Law, and Policy.* AAAS, Washington, D.C.
33. **Wivel, N. A., and L. Walters.** 1993. Germ-line gene modification and disease prevention: some medical and ethical perspectives. *Science* **262**:533–538.

Appendix I | *Class Surveys*

The following three surveys are designed for classroom use. It is recommended that students be given the responsibility for administering the surveys and compiling results. Assigned students should present the results and lead class discussion. Surveys 1 and 2 cover general areas. Survey 3 corresponds to Chapter 2.

Survey 1: Survey of Research Trainees
General Information

1. Are you currently a graduate student?   yes   no

2. Are you a classified staff person?   yes   no

3. Are you a faculty member, postdoctoral worker, or research assistant?   yes   no

4. Are you currently registered in or have you taken a course in scientific integrity?   yes   no

5. Do you hold a first professional degree? (MD, DDS, Pharm D, Bach. Pharmacy, Bach. Nursing)   yes   no

6. Are you currently involved in a research project?   yes   no

7. After your training program do you plan to continue with an academic career?   yes   no

8. Have you taken any other course on the ethics of scientific investigation?   yes   no

9. Have you had discussions with a scientific mentor on these issues?   yes   no

10. Have you been an author of a published paper or abstract?   yes   no

Ethical Issues

11. Have you been an author on a paper for which any of the authors had not made a sufficient contribution to warrant credit for the work?   yes   no

12. Has your name been omitted from a paper for which you made a substantial contribution?   yes   no

13. Do you have firsthand knowledge of scientists intentionally altering or fabricating data for the purpose of publication?   yes   no

14. Since entering a college/university have you cheated to improve a test grade?   yes   no

15. Since entering a college/university have you modified research or experimental results to improve the outcome?   yes   no

16. Since entering a college/university have you reported research or experimental results which you knew to be untrue?   yes   no

17. Since entering a college/university have you plagiarized the work of someone else?   yes   no

18. If it would expedite publication of your work, would you be willing to fabricate data?   yes   no

19. If it would expedite publication of your work, would you be willing to select or omit data to fit your hypothesis?   yes   no

20. If it would enhance a grant application, would you be willing to fabricate data?   yes   no

21. If it would enhance a grant application, would you be willing to select or omit data to fit your hypothesis?   yes   no

Data Access and Sharing

22. Have you ever received the advice that sharing of research data constitutes good science?   yes   no

In general, *before publication,* would you be willing to share your results with:

23. —a colleague from your department?   yes   no

24. —a member of another department at your university?   yes   no

25. —a scientist from another university?   yes   no

26. —a friend who is also working in your field of research?   yes   no

27. —a competitor in your field of research?   yes   no

As far as you know, who has final approval as to what will be done with your data (research notebooks, details of methods, raw data)?

28. —you	yes	no
29. —your mentor, principal investigator of project	yes	no
30. —the granting agency	yes	no
31. —the university	yes	no
32. —don't know	yes	no

At what time should research data reasonably be made available to anyone who requests them?

33. —while the project is in progress?	yes	no
34. —when data collection is complete?	yes	no
35. —when data analysis is complete?	yes	no
36. —when the manuscript has been written?	yes	no
37. —when the manuscript has been accepted for publication?	yes	no
38. —when the paper is published?	yes	no
39. Would you report a coworker who you believe has violated scientific integrity standards?	yes	no
40. Would you report your supervisor/advisor who you believe has violated scientific integrity standards?	yes	no

Adapted from: "Survey of Research Trainees at UCSD," developed by M. Kalichman, 1990. Used with permission. See: Kalichman, M. W., and P. J.

Friedman. 1992. A pilot study of biomedical trainees' perceptions concerning research ethics. *Acad. Med.* **67**:769–775.

Survey 2: Perceptions on the Incidence of Scientific Misconduct

The perception of increased incidence of scientific misconduct in recent times has been discussed in varying contexts. Indicate the degree to which you agree or disagree with the following observations as potential contributing factors to scientific misconduct. Use the following numerical scale to indicate your feelings.

Strongly agree	1
Agree	2
Disagree	3
Strongly disagree	4

1. Change in the quality (investigative vs. factual reporting) and quantity of all types of news reporting.

2. Increased number of practicing scientists and scientific trainees.

3. Increased scientific and public focus on scientists and research groups working in "hot" areas.

4. Increased number of very large, but poorly managed, research groups.

5. Lack of lay public understanding of the scientific process.

6. Increased competition for research funds.

7. Increased emphasis in academic institutions on scholarly productivity being necessary for the attainment of promotion and tenure.

8. Growing necessity for collaborative work to pursue many problems in the biomedical sciences; division of labor precludes all participating investigators from having scientific competence in the theory and techniques being used.

9. Competition to rapidly publish in prestigious journals in order to keep research programs viable.

10. Increased numbers of scientific journals, especially those published by for-profit entities (rather than societies).

11. Increased manifestation of multicultural differences and values in scientists and scientific trainees working together in the same environment.

12. Scientists' fear of admitting honest error after research results are formally reported.

13. Attitude that even if data suffer from honest error their publication will result in correction by other workers.

14. Inadequacies in the peer review systems for grants and research articles.

15. Proliferation of essentially non-peer-reviewed publications (e.g., meeting monographs).

16. Attitudes deriving from the increased amount of "nonpublic domain" or "confidential" research being done in industry and in government.

17. Increased complexity of biomedical scientific research makes repeating work time consuming, expensive, and laborious.

18. The discharge of mentoring responsibilities varies greatly in the profession and this results in the uneven education and socialization of research trainees.

Survey 3: Predoctoral Mentoring

Indicate the degree to which you agree or disagree with the following issues related to the duties and responsibilities of predoctoral mentoring.

Strongly agree   1
Agree   2
Disagree   3
Strongly disagree   4

1. Prior to accepting trainees into their laboratories, mentors must be prepared to financially support all aspects of the advisee's graduate training (stipend, tuition and fees, all research expenses, travel).

2. Mentors should not accept a trainee into their laboratory without the student first spending a brief rotation period working at the bench in that laboratory.

3. Mentors should consider the following in deciding on whether to accept a potential trainee in their laboratories:

    A. academic performance prior to graduate school

    B. academic performance in graduate school

    C. motivation

    D. personality, especially in regard to the trainee's interaction with other lab members

    E. recommendations from teachers or colleagues who have know the potential trainee

4. Mentors should set a limit to the number of trainees they accept into their laboratories; this limit should be based on financial and physical resources as well as on supervisory considerations.

5. Mentors should set a limit to the overall size of their research groups (trainees, technicians, support personnel) based on financial and physical resources, and on supervisory and management considerations.

6. Mentors should provide specific instruction to their trainees on the organization of databooks including issues related to format, collection and recording of data, retention of data, and ownership of data.

7. Mentors should regularly check that their trainees are adhering to the laboratory standards of good record keeping.

8. Mentors and trainees together should write a detailed plan of the trainee's research goals at a very early point in the trainee's program.

9. Mentors personally should educate their trainees in all matters related to laboratory safety, use of hazardous materials (including isotopes), and good laboratory practice.

10. Mentors personally should educate their trainees in all matters related to the use of animals in research.

11. Mentors personally should educate their trainees in all matters related to the use of human subjects in research.

12. Mentors should prepare, distribute, and update as needed to supervisory and responsibility structure of their research laboratories.

13. Mentors should have a defined policy with regard to scientific publication, manuscript preparation, and authorship attribution; this should be formally communicated to advisees early in their training program.

14. Mentors should meet privately and regularly (once every seven to ten days) with each of their trainees to discuss the trainee's research progress, analyze data, plan experiments, and set goals as appropriate.

15. Mentors should hold regularly scheduled meetings of their entire research group to review individual projects.

16. Mentors should regularly talk to their trainees about the people and politics of science.

17. Mentors should encourage their trainees to present their research results at local, regional, and national meetings.

18. Mentors should financially support their trainees' participation in regional and national meetings, whether or not they present their results at such meetings.

19. Mentors should be active in introducing their trainees to other scientists (e.g., visiting seminar speakers, other scientists at meetings).

20. Mentors should involve their trainees in the preparation of grant proposals, including such activities as:

    A. presentation and analysis of raw data for inclusion in the proposal

    B. development and critique of experimental design

    C. proofreading and editing

21. Mentors should share financial information about their grants with their trainees, including:

    A. how budgets are developed

    B. periodic expenditure reports of grant funds

22. Mentors should monitor trainees closely enough so as to be able to spot behavioral changes in trainees that might indicate unusual stress of any sort.

23. Mentors should provide close supervision and counseling to trainees whom they identify as suffering from inordinate stress of any type.

24. Mentors should provide career counseling throughout the training program, but especially in the latter stages of the trainee's program.

25. Mentors should encourage healthy competition among trainees in their laboratories.

26. Mentors should explain the benefits of professional society membership to their trainees and encourage them to join appropriate societies as student members.

27. Mentors should provide critiques of any verbal scientific presentation a trainee makes.

28. Mentors should provide trainees with assistance and instruction in classroom teaching skills.

29. Mentors should provides trainees with assistance and instruction in how to write a scientific paper.

30. Mentors should provide trainees with assistance and instruction in how to read a scientific paper.

Extended Case Studies

The following cases may be used for in-class discussion or they may be used as writing assignments.

1. Definition of Scientific Misconduct (Chapter 1)

Case information

Consider the following collection of proposed and working definitions which have been forwarded (and revised) from a variety of sources. Then respond to A through D below.

From the U.S. Public Health Service, National Institutes of Health (NIH):

"Misconduct" is defined as (1) serious deviation, such as fabrication, falsification, or plagiarism, from accepted practices in carrying out research or in reporting the results of research; or (2) material failure to comply with Federal requirements affecting specific aspects of the conduct of research, e.g., the protection of human subjects and the welfare of laboratory animals. (NIH Guide for Grants and Contracts, Vol. 15, No. 11, July 18, 1986)

"Misconduct" or "Misconduct in Science" means fabrication, falsification, plagiarism, or other practices that seriously deviate from those that are commonly accepted within the scientific community for proposing, conducting, or reporting research. It does not include honest error or honest differences in interpretations or judgments of data. (Federal Register **54**:32446–32451, August 8, 1989)

Misconduct is defined as the intentional fabrication or falsification of data, research procedures or data analysis; plagiarism; and other fraudulent activ-

ities in proposing, conducting, or reporting the results of or reviewing research. (U.S. Public Health Service Advisory Committee on Scientific Integrity recommended definition on November 17, 1991)

Research fraud is defined as plagiarism, fabrication, or intentional falsification of data, research procedures or data analysis, or other deliberate misrepresentation in proposing, conducting, reporting, or reviewing research. (U.S. Public Health Service Advisory Committee on Research Integrity [committee name changed] recommended definition on March 7, 1992)

Research misconduct is defined as plagiarism, fabrication or intentional falsification of data, research procedures or data analysis, or other deliberate misrepresentation in proposing, conducting, reporting, or reviewing research. (U.S. Public Health Service, Office of Research Integrity proposed definition, October 1992)

From the National Science Foundation (NSF):

Misconduct means (1) fabrication, falsification, plagiarism, or other serious deviation from accepted practices in proposing, carrying out, or reporting results from research; (2) material failure to comply with Federal requirements for protection of researchers, human subjects, or the public or for ensuring the welfare of laboratory animals; or (3) failure to meet other material legal requirements governing research. (Federal Register **52**:24466–24470, July 1, 1987)

Misconduct means fabrication, falsification, plagiarism or other serious deviation from accepted practices in preparing, carrying out, or reporting results from activities funded by NSF, or retaliation of any kind against a person who reported or provided information about suspected or alleged misconduct and who has not acted in bad faith. (Federal Register **56**:22286–22290. May 14, 1991)

From the Federation of American Societies for Experimental Biology (FASEB) and the U.S. National Academy of Sciences (NAS):

Misconduct in science means fabrication, falsification, or plagiarism, but does not include those factors intrinsic to the process of science, such as honest error, conflicting data, or differences in interpretation or judgement of data or experimental design. (FASEB, 1990)

Misconduct in science is defined as fabrication, falsification, or plagiarism, in proposing, performing, or reporting research. Misconduct in science does not include errors of judgement; errors in the recording, selection, or analysis of data; difference in opinions involving the interpretation of data; or misconduct unrelated to the research process. (NAS, 1992)

Student assignment

A. For each of the definitions of scientific misconduct presented, discuss the following issues from your point of view:

—appropriateness of scope
—clarity; latitude for interpretation
—burden of proof: where should it reside?
—intent to deceive as the critical issue
—protection of the "whistleblower."

B. Discuss your views on the specificity of the language in the various definitions. Depending on your point of view, amend one or more definitions to conform with your thinking and defend your position.

C. Discuss the issue of inclusion of the phrase "other serious deviation" in the definition of scientific misconduct. Is this appropriate?

D. One NSF official (Chapter 1, reference 3) argues that federal funding agencies have an enforcement role that protects the integrity of the research process and its attendant funding vehicles. His central argument is that some actions must be classified as scientific misconduct irrespective of whether they are covered by general laws or regulations or whether they are unique to science and scientific research.

On the other hand, an NAS panel report (Chapter 1, reference 9) defines a category of "other misconduct" beyond that of scientific misconduct. This former category is based on arguments that actions fitting this description "(1) do not require expert knowledge to resolve these complaints and, (2) should be governed by mechanisms that apply to all institutional members, not just those who receive government research awards." The NAS panel report says that "certain forms of unacceptable behavior are clearly not unique to the conduct of science, although they may occur in a laboratory or research environment."

Using examples not considered fabrication, falsification, or plagiarism (e.g., vandalism, tampering, misuse of grant funds), defend or refute their being classified as scientific misconduct. Prepare a short hypothetical case to illustrate your point.

2. Electronic Archiving of Research Grant Results (Chapter 3)

Case information
Assume the following memo reflects a future NIH policy, then respond to A through E below.

* * *

TO: Appropriate Program Officer, NIH–NCI
FROM: Principal Investigator
RE: Final electronic report: CA 12345-05-10

Attached you will find a copy of a CD ROM diskette labelled: "CA 12345-05-10." The information contained on this diskette corresponds to my NIH grant award, "Antisense control of human leukemias." The funding period corresponds to years -05 (1 May *XXXX*) through -10 (30 April *XXXX*) of this project. A competing renewal of this program (years -11 through -15) was approved for funding earlier this year. I understand that these new funds will not be released until my attached electronic report is filed with and approved by the NIH.

The diskette contains the following information:

1. Names and up-to-date curricula vitae of all professional personnel, trainees, and technical staff who worked on the project during this reporting period.

2. All pages of all databooks and original records pertaining to this project. This includes audioadrographic films, photographs, and micrographs. Such photographic data have been cross-indexed to appropriate experiments in the various databooks. These materials were digitized and entered onto the diskette by use of a scanner and appropriate software employing "WORM" ("write once-read many") technology as prescribed by the NIH. All materials were entered on a weekly basis and were electronically dated using a digital time-stamping program. The electronic time-stamping data have been submitted to the prescribed independent vendor. The signatures of the principal investigator and the project worker(s) were also entered and dated via scanning on a weekly basis to certify the ac-

curacy and authenticity of the recorded data. Where appropriate, signatures of witnesses to certain results were scanned into the file as part of the page on which they appeared.

3. All published manuscripts and preprints of submitted or in-press manuscripts also are included on this diskette. The published papers were loaded onto this diskette by scanning and digitization. Note that one of the manuscripts contains several color photographs. These have been scanned and processed with the appropriate software so as to be reproduced electronically or in hard copy as full-color illustrations. The preprints and reprints were entered as standard word-processing files, including picture files of all manuscript figures.

4. The original grant proposal and all appendix material have been entered onto the disk using a combination of direct word-processing file transfer and scanning of all halftone and graphic materials. Also included are the progress reports for the four noncompeting renewal applications filed in connection with this grant award.

5. A file designated "Aims–Progress" is also included on this diskette. As prescribed by NIH, this file contains all original, additional, and modified Specific Aims for this project. These are cross-referenced with respect to relevant databooks and materials, or with publications associated with this project.

I understand that I am to retain a copy of this disk 15 years from the date of this memo. I further understand that NIH will retain the attached diskette indefinitely.

Student assignment

A. Is such an electronic filing likely to have an effect on the incidence or occurrence of scientific fraud? Can you envision it deterring fraud in science? If so, how? If not, why not? In presenting your arguments, consider the effects on two kinds of personalities: the unintentional self-deceiver and the deliberate perpetrator of fraud.

B. Can such a system create a situation(s) that could lead to even more kinds of scientific fraud? Explain.

C. Who should have access to this information, under what conditions and by what means? Defend your answer.

D. What implications would such a reporting system have for requests made under the Freedom of Information Act? (see Chapter 8)

E. What implications would such a reporting system have for invention disclosures and for the filing of patents? (see Chapter 8)

3. Blastomere Analysis before Implantation (Chapter 9)

Case information

You practice in a large *in vitro* fertilization clinic, where blastomere analysis before implantation (BABI) is offered. A couple seeking *in vitro* fertilization requests that an "embryo biopsy" be done because each is a Tay-Sachs carrier. Determination of whether or not the embryo will have Tay-Sachs does not require determination of the embryo's sex. However, the wife states, "This may be our only chance to have a child, and we both want a boy. Check the sex of the embryos, and don't implant any female embryos!"

Student assignment

A. What will you say to the couple, and how will you determine which embryos to implant?

B. Is selection against male embryos on the basis of potential sex-linked genetic abnormalities different from selection against female embryos on the basis of cultural biases?

C. If the care provider and recipients differ in their stances on sex selection, should the final decision about sex selection be guided by the ethical base of the care provider or of the recipient?

D. Selection of embryos on the basis of sex is not considered unethical by some contemporary scholars. (However, it is prohibited under the German Embryo Protection Act of October 24, 1990.) Should the religious affiliation of the couple influence the final decision?

E. More generally, who should control what tests will be run on the embryos and which embryos will be selected for implantation? Does the fact that recipients are paying for the service influence the criteria for selection of embryos? How much input should researchers, care providers, potential parents, legislators, and society in general have in determining what is an acceptable implant?

F. Does BABI differ from amniocentesis? If so, how? Does BABI differ from infanticide? If so, how?

4. Authorship, Peer Review, and Sharing Data
(Chapters 4 and 8)

Case information

You are the editor-in-chief of a molecular biology journal. Twelve associate editors comprise your editorial board. They receive papers directly and oversee the *ad hoc* peer review of these submitted manuscripts. You receive a letter from one of your associate editors asking you for advice on how he should handle a problem. The details of this issue are as follows:

1. A manuscript handled by the associate editor (Dr. Red) has been in print for about six months.

2. Dr. White is the corresponding author and the head of the lab that submitted the paper. Dr. White was contacted in writing by Dr. Blue requesting a series of recombinant plasmids carrying sequences of a newly discovered herpes-like virus which infects and transforms mouse cells. The published manuscript carefully details the uniqueness of the virus using biological techniques and nucleic acid hybridization studies.

3. Dr. Blue, an expert DNA virologist, informs Dr. White that he wants to use the viral fragments to do complementation experiments with a specific group of viruses.

4. Dr. White writes back to Dr. Blue telling him that those experiments have already been done in his own lab and the results were negative (but not published).

5. Dr. Blue then writes to Dr. White again, requesting the same recombinant plasmids. He argues that Dr. White's reason is not an appropriate one and that Dr. White is interfering with his right to confirm and verify results in the published literature.

6. Dr. White responds by letter to Dr. Blue strongly stating that he is only obliged to release such materials when the requestor provides reasonable disclosure of intended use. He accuses Dr. Blue of seeking these materials to advance his re-

search in areas that will directly compete with Dr. White's program. Under the circumstances, Dr. White argues, this is both unfair and unethical.

7. The policy of the journal with respect to sharing of materials reads as follows: "Publication of original research reports in this journal indicates that the authors are willing to make available and distribute clones of cells or DNA molecules, antibodies, or other similar materials to interested researchers associated with academic or not-for-profit institutions. The authors may reserve the right to limit quantities of such distributed material. Materials requested must have been used in the experiments reported in the published paper."

8. Dr. Red, the associate editor, asks you as editor-in-chief to handle this situation. Dr. Red asks you to write him with advice and a suggested course of action.

Student assignment

Compose a requested letter to Dr. Red. Include the following in your letter:

A. Your perspective on this series of events.

B. Any additional questions you'd like to have answered by Dr. White or Dr. Blue.

C. Your suggested course of action. If you suggest that either Dr. White or Dr. Blue be contacted in writing, be explicit as to what information should be in the letter(s).

5. Sharing Research Materials (Chapters 4 and 8)

Case information

You are an NIH-funded university faculty member who writes to an investigator requesting a recombinant plasmid that carries a gene encoding a major surface protein of a human pathogenic bacterium. Your letter precisely spells out your plans for using this recombinant plasmid in your research project. This surface protein gene has been cloned by the investigator and its cloning has been reported in the peer-reviewed literature. The investigator is a staff scientist at a private research institute. You get a prompt response to your request in the form of a letter from the research administrator of the institute. The letter describes the terms under which a bacterial strain containing the requested recombinant plasmid (referred to in the letter as "the material") will be released to you. The letter contains language that pertains to your use of the material being requested. A list of the issues covered includes:

1. The material must not be administered to humans.

2. The material is being provided only for the stated use; permission must be sought from the research institute if other uses of the material are planned.

3. The material may not be released to any other investigators outside of the faculty member's lab.

4. You must provide the names of any lab staff or trainees working with the material.

5. You certify that you will not hold the research institute legally responsible for any harm or injury that may be caused by the material or its use.

6. You cannot disclose, by any means, any of the work you do with this material without first seeking and obtaining the permission of the research institute.

7. You cannot use the material for any commercial or profit-making purposes.

8. The research institute will be granted an option for exclusive licensing of any inventions coming from the planned work with this material. The license will be negotiated in good faith between you and the research institute.

9. At the conclusion of the work the material will be returned to the research institute or destroyed.

10. All lab members must be notified in writing of the terms of the release of the material and its use under those terms.

You are asked to countersign this letter and return it to the research institute before the recombinant plasmid can be released to you. This is your first experience with such a letter. You do have some concerns about certain of the items that it contains.

You show the letter to a colleague, who comments that such agreements aren't legally worth the paper they're printed on. He advises you to just sign it and return it so you can get the plasmid and move ahead with your work.

You show the letter to your departmental chair, who informs you that the letter must be countersigned by someone authorized to sign on behalf of your university, in this case the director of sponsored programs.

You show the letter to another faculty colleague, who confirms your notions that some of the clauses are too restrictive and inappropriate according to current standards of exchange of biological materials. He recommends that you send the letter back suggesting the deletion or modification of such clauses.

Student assignment
Comment on the advice being given by each of these individuals. What, if any, clauses are unacceptable to you? Why? Where might you find "current standards of exchange of biological materials" if such standards really exist? Finally, explain the course of action you would take in this situation.

6. Conflict of Conscience (Chapters 5 and 7)

Case information
You are chair of an institutional advisory committee on the care and use of laboratory animals. This committee reviews and recommends policies and practices on the use of laboratory animals, and reviews experimental protocols prepared by investigators. It consists of nine faculty, two members outside the institution, and you as chair. One-third of the faculty members rotate off the committee each year. A professor in a basic science department asks you to nominate him for membership on the committee. Some salient points are as follows:

1. The basic science professor is a theoretical biologist who is internationally known for his computer simulations.

2. The professor has testified before legislative bodies opposing the use of pets in research.

3. The professor has known associations with members of a militant animal rights and animal liberation group.

4. The professor has been very active in developing computer-assisted instructional materials.

5. The professor has been very active in university governance.

6. Your institution has a nationally accredited laboratory animal facility managed by a team of veterinarians and trained animal care workers.

7. The faculty of your institution has a number of extramurally funded research projects using rodents, rabbits, cats, dogs, and primates.

8. The extramurally funded research is sponsored by private agencies, federal agencies, and private industry.

9. The animal research comprises studies in nutrition, immunology, drug testing, biochemistry, neurology, toxicology, infectious diseases, and chemical dependency.

Student assignment

You discuss this with the senior administrator for research, who appoints the membership of this committee. She asks you to make a decision based upon your best judgment and to

1. Write a letter to her, advising her of your recommendation, along with reasons for your decision.

2. Write a letter to the professor who asked you to nominate him for committee membership, giving your decision and reasons for your decision.

3. Prepare a draft of your response should members of the institutional advisory committee ask you about the matter.

4. Prepare a draft of your plan of action should a member of the press or an animal rights organization ask you about the matter.

7. Conflict of Effort (Chapters 2 and 7)

Case information

You are chair of a renowned chemistry department in a major research-intensive university. One of your outstanding professors is sought after as a member of advisory panels, lecturer, consultant, and leader in professional organizations. This professor continues to publish and accept assignments as coordinator of formal courses. During the past year, you have received complaints and overheard comments that he is missing departmental committee meetings and is frequently not prepared to make scheduled presentations. Upon inquiry, you discover the following:

1. The professor is advisor to two graduate students, two postdoctoral research trainees, and three technicians.

2. One graduate student is supervised by a postdoctoral research trainee, who also supervises one of the technicians.

3. The other graduate student and postdoctoral research trainee each supervise one technician.

4. The professor is on an international commission that meets overseas a total of 15 working days per year.

5. The professor has established a consulting company, which he operates from a home office.

6. The professor makes 12 consulting visits per year.

7. The professor is president of a national professional society that requires that he spend 24 days per year at the society's meetings or at its headquarters.

8. The professor is on a grant review panel that meets nine days per year.

9. The professor is editor-in-chief of a professional journal. He attends meetings with the publisher six days per year, and spends approximately one hour each day on editorial matters.

10. The professor is on the editorial board of another professional journal and reviews about two dozen manuscripts per year.

11. The professor attends two professional meetings each year, each four days long.

12. The professor gives one lecture each month at another institution.

13. The professor is asked to testify before legislative committees and regulatory panels a total of six days per year.

14. The professor has assigned his two postdoctoral workers to present 30 hours of his assigned 45 hours of lectures.

15. The professor frequently misses departmental and institutional committee meetings.

Student assignment
Compose an annual letter of evaluation of this professor, addressing these issues:

1. Activities to be encouraged

2. Activities to be discouraged

3. Other advice

4. Overall evaluation

8. Conflict of Interest (Chapter 7)

Case information
You are chair of a department in an academic health sciences center. You have recruited a faculty member whose spouse has a master's

degree in the same field. The faculty member has applied for a grant from a federal agency and has just received an award notice. The faculty member comes to you to establish a research assistant position on the grant. She indicates that she plans to hire her spouse for this position. Some salient points follow:

1. The faculty member and spouse worked together to collect preliminary data. The spouse worked as an unpaid volunteer.

2. The faculty member and spouse both contributed to the preparation of the grant application, in which the faculty member was named as the principal investigator and the spouse was named as the research assistant.

3. The faculty member and spouse maintain different professional names.

4. The thesis work of the spouse directly relates to the goals and methods described in the grant.

5. The faculty member and the spouse have established that they can work together effectively on this project, so there would be no delay in pursuing the grant.

6. The faculty member and the spouse have published a preliminary report as coauthors.

Student assignment

You discuss this matter with the personnel officer of the academic health sciences center. Several issues are raised, and you are asked to write a memorandum to the faculty member and one to the personnel officer, giving your recommended action and the reasons for your decision. The issues to be addressed include:

1. Does this constitute preselection of a job candidate, thereby violating the academic health sciences center's commitment to equal employment opportunity?

2. Does this involve direct supervision of a member of the immediate family and thereby violate the academic health sciences center's antinepotism rules?

3. Is this an acceptable or desirable arrangement, and if so, how can the arrangement be set up to meet legal requirements?

4. Are there additional issues that might arise in the future that should be resolved at this time; for example, supervision of graduate students or additional technicians?

9. Publication of Data (Chapters 3 and 4)

Case information

A postdoctoral presented her research results at an informal laboratory meeting. Her work involved the molecular cloning of a relatively large genomic fragment isolated from a bacterium. A gene encoding a 200-kDa protein has been mapped on this genomic fragment. The entire fragment was cloned in a bacteriophage lambda vector and is approximately 20 kb in size. The gene in question carried by this fragment has been sequenced and its gene product has been biochemically characterized. There is some reason to believe that this gene is part of an operon. The postdoctoral indicates that this portion of the work including the sequencing and characterization of the gene product is in advanced draft form for submission to a peer-reviewed journal. The 20-kb lambda insert consists of seven smaller restriction fragments, all of which have been subcloned with the exception of a 2-kb fragment at one of the termini of the original insert. The draft manuscript focuses heavily on the cloning of the 200-kDa protein gene, its mapping on the 20-kb insert, and its sequence determination. The postdoctoral points out that the original lambda clone carrying the 20-kb insert has been lost. The only sample of the recombinant phage that was being stored for future use no longer gives rise to phage plaques. She contends that this is not a significant issue in relation to the manuscript as most of the fragment has been subcloned and that all the clones involving the 200-kDa protein gene are available as plasmid subclones. A discussion among the group members subsequently ensues regarding the handling of this situation. The laboratory head actively solicits the opinions of some of the individuals (all of whom are postdoctorals) seated around the table.

Gene Jones suggests that the paper describe the original lambda phage clone and not mention that the clone has been lost. Since 90% of the original clone is available as subcloned fragments, Dr. Jones contends that the point is moot and that there is no need to mention the status of the original clone.

Bill Thomas suggests a modification for Dr. Jones's proposal. He proposes that the missing restriction fragment be isolated from a plasmid library of the organism. This would be far easier than attempting to reclone the entire 20-kb fragment. The cloning of the missing fragment would thus result in the entire 20-kb sequence being available and would preclude problems with supplying any of the fragments of the original clone to other interested investigators. Accordingly, Dr. Thomas argues that with this goal accomplished there won't be any need to mention that the original phage clone is no longer available. He argues that in practice, his solution makes the entire 20-kb available in an appropriate context.

Gail Smith suggests that the manuscript be submitted as soon as possible but that the paper be modified to disclose that the original phage clone is no longer available. She suggests that the clone can be described and its map presented based on experiments that have been performed, but an indication that the clone is not presently available in the laboratory should be made in the manuscript. Since the subclones of the sequenced and genetically characterized area are available, Dr. Smith contends that this solution is practical and is not likely to lead to confusion or to possible misinterpretation in terms of what is being presented in the paper.

Don Williams states that if the original phage clone is to be described in the paper, it must be available. Accordingly, he argues strongly that the clone must be reisolated and present in the laboratory stock collection before the paper can be submitted.

Kathy Steward favors the idea forwarded by Dr. Williams but suggests that the paper be submitted before the clone is available. The paper is likely to be returned with reviewers' comments, and submission of a revised manuscript can always be delayed at that point if the clone is still not available (which, she contends, is not very likely).

Student assignment
Imagine that you are the laboratory supervisor at this meeting. Respond to the various arguments being presented by these postdoctor-

als. What proposed solutions or combination of solutions will you embrace as being acceptable? What acceptable solutions of your own, if any, do you have to offer?

Appendix III | *Standards of Conduct*

A collection of guidelines for the conduct of research, specific research policies and practices, and policies and procedures for handling of misconduct may be found in a monograph published in 1993 by the U.S. National Academy of Sciences: *Responsible Science* (Vol. II). *Ensuring the Integrity of the Research Process*. National Academy Press, 2101 Constitution Avenue, N.W., Washington, D.C. 20418.

The following provides general information on the location of other written documents that deal with standards of conduct in the research and academic settings.

Federal Agency Documents. These documents are concerned with such things as procedures and regulations related to the identification and prosecution of scientific misconduct. They also deal with other specific issues related to scientific integrity and responsible conduct. They are usually available at the institutional level, or can be found directly in the *Federal Register* or the *NIH Guide for Grants and Contracts.* Often the issues presented are under discussion and subsequent ongoing publication will occur. When rules are finally established, the phrase "Final Rule" is included in the title of the article. These documents usually reflect the activities and authority of the Office of Research Integrity of the U.S. Public Health Service (for the National Institutes of Health [NIH]) or the Office of the Inspector General of the National Science Foundation (NSF). These publications may be found in libraries or in institutionally sponsored program offices (often called "grants offices"). Frequently, individual investigators receive the *NIH Guide for Grants and Contracts* by subscription. This communication is now distributed electronically and can be accessed by individuals and institutions. Check with your office of sponsored programs on where you can locate your institutional copy.

269

Two important announcements have been published after *Responsible Science*. They are the NSF's notice: "Investigator Financial Disclosure Policy" (*Federal Register* **59** [No. 123]:33308–33312, June 28, 1994) and the Department of Health and Human Services proposed rules: "Objectivity in Research" (*Federal Register* **59** [No. 123]:33242–33251, June 28, 1994). The NSF's revised requirements for submission of proposals have an effective implementation date of June 28, 1995. The revised award conditions require institutions to maintain written and enforced policies on investigator conflicts of interest. The U.S. Public Health Service (USPHS) proposed rules are supposed to be consistent with NSF rules and are expected to be implemented at about the same time. The USPHS proposed rules require that institutions that apply to them for research funds assume responsibility for ensuring that financial interests of the institution's employees do not compromise the objectivity with which the sponsored research is designed, conducted, or reported. It is anticipated that these policies will be extended to other federal agencies and will undergo further revisions to reduce inconsistencies.

Federal and Institutional Guidelines for the Use and Protection of Human Research Subjects and of Animals. These documents can usually be located at institutional sponsored programs offices or the institutional offices of the federally mandated Investigational Review Board. Federal guidelines prevail, but special institutional guidelines may augment or supplement them.

Appropriate Professional Society Code of Ethics or Standards for Scientific Conduct. Professional scientific societies have conduct and ethics codes, which may be published from time to time, usually in society-sponsored journals or publications. The central administrative offices of the relevant society may be contacted to get these documents.

Institutional Policies Document for Conduct of Research. A growing number of academic and research institutions have developed policy documents dealing with the responsible conduct of research. Your institution may not have one yet or may be in the process of developing one. Check with your sponsored programs office to see what exists at your institution. Specific examples such documents are found in *Responsible Science,* Vol. II.

Institutional Computer Ethics Policy. Academic and research institutions often have policies on the ethical use of computers and, especially, computer software. Central computer support offices at academic and research institutions will have such documents.

Institutional Documents Discussing Copyright Issues, Intellectual Property, and Conflict of Interest. These documents are usually distributed periodically to faculty but also can be obtained from offices of sponsored programs, the vice president's or provost's office, or the office of the institutional legal counsel.

Worker's Right to Know and Hazard Communication Documentation. Such documents are sent to faculty periodically, but they can also be obtained from the institutional safety office. Mentors and laboratory heads have certain legal requirements imposed upon them regarding the regulation of practices and the communication of potentially hazardous materials and situations to all of their laboratory personnel.

Institutional Academic Honor Code Document. Honor code documents usually are distributed to graduate students upon matriculation into their programs. They can be obtained from the office of the academic dean or the dean of students.

Guidelines for Scholarly Publication. Scientific journals regularly publish guidelines for contributors. These can appear in every issue of the publication; often they appear at the beginning or end of volume sequences or at the beginning or end of the calendar year. Such guidelines vary in scope and content and may cover such things as authorship attribution, sharing of research materials, conflict of interest disclosure, and communication of results to the media prior to acceptance (see Chapter 4). Investigators should be familiar with the publication guidelines of any journal to which they intend to submit a scientific manuscript.

Index

postdoctoral, relationship with
mentor, case study, 36–37
predoctoral, expectations for, 29–32
reproduction of each other's
work, case study, 38
respect for mentor, 19–20
responsibilities regarding animal
rights, case study, 128
romantic relationship in
laboratory
views of, case study, 34–35
with mentor, case study, 37–38
survey of, 241–245
training, mentor's views of, case
study, 38–39
trust in mentor, 20–21
working hours, case study, 35
Trainee-mentor relationship. *See*
Mentor-trainee relationship
Trust, in mentor-trainee relationship,
20–21

U
Universities and conflict of interest,
174–175
Unpublished information cited in
manuscripts, instructions to
authors regarding, 75–76

U.S. Public Health Service (USPHS),
data ownership guidelines,
45–47
Utilitarianism
in animal experimentation, 104–106
criticism of, 105–106
described, 104
Singer's, and animal "rights,"
106–108

V
Victorian antivivisectionist
movement, history, 123–124

W
"Whistleblower," 5
Witness databook, 58–60
*Worker's Right to Know and Hazard
Communication Documentation,*
271
Working hours, standard for
trainees, case study, 35
World Medical Association
Declaration of Helsinki, 156–160
Writing the Laboratory Notebook, 42